End-of-Life Decision Making

Basic Bioethics

Glenn McGee and Arthur Caplan, editors

End-of-Life Decision Making

A Cross-National Study

Robert H. Blank and Janna C. Merrick

The MIT Press
Cambridge, Massachusetts
London, England

© 2005 Massachusetts Institute of Technology

All rights reserved. No part of this book may be reproduced in any form by any electronic or mechanical means (including photocopying, recording, or information storage and retrieval) without permission in writing from the publisher.

MIT Press books may be purchased at special quantity discounts for business or sales promotional use. For information, please email special_sales@mitpress.mit.edu or write to Special Sales Department, The MIT Press, 5 Cambridge Center, Cambridge, MA 02142.

This book was set in Sabon on 3B2 by Asco Typesetters, Hong Kong and was printed and bound in the United States of America.

Library of Congress Cataloging-in-Publication Data

End-of-life decision making : a cross-national study / [edited by] Robert H. Blank and Janna C. Merrick.
    p.   cm. — (Basic bioethics)
Includes bibliographical references and index.
ISBN 0-262-02574-4 (hbk. : alk. paper)
1. Terminal care—Cross-cultural studies. 2. Palliative treatment—Cross-cultural studies. 3. Medical policy—Cross-cultural studies. 4. Death—Cross-cultural studies. I. Blank, Robert H. II. Merrick, Janna C. III. Series.
R726.8.E534   2005
352.17′5—dc22   2004053084

10 9 8 7 6 5 4 3 2

For Marty Gladding, who walked her final journey with optimism, faith and love

Contents

Series Foreword

We are pleased to present the fourteenth book in the series Basic Bioethics. The series presents innovative works in bioethics to a broad audience and introduces seminal scholarly manuscripts, state-of-the-art reference works, and textbooks. Such broad areas as the philosophy of medicine, advancing genetics and biotechnology, end-of-life care, health and social policy, and the empirical study of biomedical life are covered.

Glenn McGee
Arthur Caplan

Basic Bioethics Series Editorial Board
Tod S. Chambers
Susan Dorr Goold
Mark Kuczewski
Herman Saatkamp

Preface

This book examines decision making that affects end-of-life or "death-related" issues in twelve disparate countries selected from among developed and developing nations. The goal is to offer a broader perspective on this topic than is normally provided in order to study the differences and similarities of ethics and policy making on end-of-life decisions across cultures. To do this, top scholars and/or practitioners in each of these countries were asked to analyze end-of-life decision making in their own country. For many of these countries, the chapters presented here are the first systematic attempt to do this, and some like China, Kenya, and Turkey, are groundbreaking studies. Some of the chapters include original data; all of them summarize existing governmental activities and cases and the current state of dying in their countries. This book should serve as a reference work on the status of death-related policies in these individual countries and a starting point for a more systematic comparative analysis of end-of-life policy making and health policy in general. It also demonstrates the tenuous nature of bioethics across these countries and the wide gap between wealthy and poor nations when it comes to these issues.

The editors would like to thank all the authors who in some cases spent innumerable hours attempting to track down data on dying that did not exist. Each of the chapters stands alone as a unique, authoritative study. The editors especially would like to thank Ole Döring, who was instrumental in arranging and preparing the chapters on China and Taiwan. We would also like to thank Clay Morgan and Art Caplan for their support and encouragement of this project and the reviewers for their invaluable comments.

End-of-Life Decision Making

1

Introduction: Issues at the End of Life

Robert H. Blank

Until recent decades, death and the dying process were largely a matter of private decisions made within specific religious and cultural frameworks. Increasingly, however, questions of how societies make decisions about the ending of life have become a matter of public policy and of ethical debate. Advances in medicine have the capacity to extend life indefinitely, but often with poor quality and escalating dependence on medical technologies. Demographically, the aging populations in most developed countries and the increasing incidence of AIDS and other chronic diseases in developing countries promise to complicate end-of-life decision making in the coming decades. As a growing proportion of societal resources are concentrated at the end of people's lives, the ethical and policy issues are bound to intensify. Thus, the more we can understand and debate the issues now, the better the chance we will have of dealing with their mounting consequences for all countries.

The literature on treatment of terminal patients, euthanasia, brain death, and other issues related to dying has expanded significantly in recent decades (for example, see Webb et al. 1997; Olick 2001; Wijdicks 2001). There remains, however, a paucity of publications on how these issues are handled across countries. Furthermore, the few cross-national studies that have been published usually include only several countries, particularly Western ones (e.g., Sass et al. 1998). This book brings together policy experts from a wide array of countries in all regions of the world to examine how these countries are coping with end-of-life issues. How are the issues defined? What is the level of debate? How are terminally ill patients treated by their respective health care systems? In light of demographic patterns, increasingly scarce health care resources, and an expanding array of lifesaving technologies, decisions affecting the end of life are becoming problematic matters of public and thus scholarly concern in most countries.

Issues Surrounding End-of-Life Decision Making

There are numerous multidimensional issues that together define the context of policy making on end-of-life issues. Although most attention in the West has focused on the elderly as terminal patients, in some countries the major focus might be on younger adult AIDS patients or on children dying from malnutrition or infectious diseases. Another important category of cases, although much smaller in number, consists of critically ill or extremely low birth-weight babies. In each of these categories, the responses to the problems they present can vary significantly across countries. Basic questions relate to what institutional services exist for care of the terminally ill; how, where, and by whom these patients are treated; how aggressive and costly the treatment regime is (e.g., the availability of intensive care units); who makes the final decisions as to level of care given; and who pays the escalating costs of dying.

More specific questions relate to the availability of medical specialists and adequate pain management, palliative care, and hospice services. The World Health Organization defines palliative care as

the active total care of patients whose disease is not responsive to curative treatment. Control of pain, of other symptoms, and of psychological, social and spiritual problems is paramount. The goal of palliative care is the achievement of the best possible quality of life for patients and their families. (World Health Organization 2002: 1)

According to the Center to Advance Palliative Care, a national initiative supported by the Robert Wood Johnson Foundation at Mount Sinai School of Medicine in New York, hospice care is an organized program for delivering palliative care. Hospice care may be provided in either a facility or the home, but the basic concept is one of comprehensive care for the dying. Although the physical facilities may be very extensive or quite minimal, according to the American Academy of Family Physicians (2003) it should include control of pain and other symptoms, psychosocial support for both the patient and family, medical services commensurate with the needs of the patient, and specially trained personnel with expertise in care of the dying and their families. What types of hospices operate and what level of palliative care and pain management are accessible to the dying in different countries?

Conversely, what, if any, boundaries or cutoff points exist for aggressive treatment of a particular category of patient, whether an extremely premature infant, an end-stage AIDS patient, or a terminally ill elderly patient? Also, where do individuals generally die? In intensive care units, hospital wards, nursing homes, hospices, or at home? Moreover, who funds this care and who ultimately makes the life-ending decision in cases where the patient is unable to so? Doctors, the family, ethics committees, the government, or some or all of these?

Accompanying the medical dimensions of policy making for the end of life are the social and legal aspects. In some Western countries, considerable emphasis in recent decades has been directed toward empowerment of the patient or patient autonomy. A wide variety of legal mechanisms have been created toward this end. Prominent among these advance directives are the living will and the durable power of attorney. The goal of advance directives is to return to the individual the ability to control the dying process, primarily by refusing life-extending interventions. However, they also contain a resource allocation dimension and in virtually all cases are designed to specify limits on continued treatment and expenditures; they are not a demand for extended intervention.

Related to advance directives are various policy initiatives and debates over the concept of euthanasia, itself loaded with complex and varied meanings both within and across cultures and countries. Some commentators distinguish between passive and active; voluntary and involuntary; and other categories of euthanasia, thus allowing for support of some but not other types (table 1.1). Others argue that such distinctions are artificial and that all forms of euthanasia are morally wrong and thus must be outlawed. Still others argue that the distinctions are of little help and that individuals should not be precluded by law or moral codes from making their own choice as to how and when to die. Although the most vehement opposition to euthanasia tends to center on those cases where the active assistance of a third party is required, the debate over doctor-assisted suicide frequently is deliberately linked with cases involving the

Table 1.1
Categories of euthanasia

	Passive Omission of measure to prolong life	*Active* Direct inducement of death
Voluntary With patient's express and informed consent.	*Passive Voluntary* Conscious *and* rational patient refuses life-prolonging treatment and request is granted.	*Active Voluntary* Conscious *and* rational patient requests and is given lethal injection.
Speculative Without express and informed consent (i.e., comatose patient, infant, dementia patient).	*Passive Speculative* Cessation of life-prolonging treatment for patient unable to give informed consent.	*Active Speculative* Lethal injection administered to patient unable to give informed consent.
Involuntary Against the express directions of the patient.	*Passive Involuntary* Cessation of life-prolonging treatment of conscious and rational person against his or her will.	*Active Involuntary* Lethal injections administered to conscious and rational patient against his or her will.

Source: Blank (1995: 163).

withholding or withdrawing of treatment, thus again clouding the lines between passive and active types of euthanasia. The question remains as to how different countries define and deal with euthanasia.

Another challenging issue is how we define the death of a human being. In response to the development of life-sustaining technologies and the need for organs for transplantation, some countries have moved to a legal definition of death as brain death. There are two critical dimensions to this issue. The first is the conceptual interpretation of what death means in the context of medical technology, since the traditional understanding of death as the irreversible cessation of cardiopulmonary functions can be "clouded by technological means of prolonging those functions in patients" (Weir 1989: 292). The second dimension centers on the appropriate clinical tests to be used to determine that a patient is in fact dead, especially when the patient's life has been prolonged by technological means. Because technologies in both of these areas are advancing rapidly (in the first instance, life-sustaining technologies and in the second, diagnostic technologies that indicate the presence or absence of specific types of activity in particular regions of the brain), and because of the linkage of brain death to the availability of organs for transplantation, the definition of death has become a contentious issue, and one that is likely to vary from country to country.

A broad array of end-of-life issues, therefore, from how and where the dying are treated, to who makes the decision to withhold or abate treatment or allow physician-assisted suicide, and to how we define and measure death elicit considerable public and professional debate. This is not surprising because decisions on the ending of life are among the most intensely emotional and ethically charged issues. Critical to understanding these issues in a broad sense is the extent to which they are common across nations and cultures or, contrarily, vary from one country to the next.

This book is an attempt to provide a foundation for more in-depth study of the issues by placing end-of-life decision making in a comparative context. Although it is dangerous to uncritically apply policies that appear to work in one country to another country, cross-national research is useful in expanding the range of options open to policy makers and in allowing them to explore the experiences of their counterparts in other jurisdictions in dealing with similar problems. Ovretveit (1998), for instance, argues that travel and information systems are making it both easier and more necessary to understand cultural and national differences. Likewise, Harrop suggests that "by examining policies comparatively, we can discover how countries vary in the policies they adopt, gain insight into why these differences exist, and identify some of the conditions under which policies succeed or fail" (1992: 3).

Comparative studies also give us cross-cultural insights as to what works or does not work in a wide variety of institutional and value contexts. Why do factors that might be viewed as overpowering in one national context, such as the attitudes of the citizens or the medical profession, result in different outcomes elsewhere? According to Immergut, the "comparative perspective shows that some factors are neither as unique nor as critical as they appear, whereas others stand out as truly significant" (Immergut 1992: 9). Ham (1997) adds that an examination of international experience is useful in demonstrating the difficulties faced by and the wide range of approaches available to policy makers. Given the complexity of these issues, only knowledge of what is happening in many countries can generate the evidence necessary to consider the full array of options.

Studying the issues across many country settings can also illuminate the commonalities of problems and variables across countries. Although at some level policy surrounding the end of life might be unique to each country, one cannot ignore the globalization of problems and potential solutions. Immediate transmission of knowledge about new medical technologies through the mass media raises public and professional expectations and demands for access to those innovations. Through the Internet, people can become informed about the newest treatments available elsewhere in the world, and public demands for them can rise accordingly. Citizens can also shop across national boundaries to determine where certain practices, such as doctor-assisted suicide, are legal. Likewise, international medical conferences and journals transfer technologies and knowledge quickly from one side of the globe to the other, thus working to globalize professional standards.

Some observers argue that these global forces reinforce the convergence theory, which posits that as countries industrialize they tend to converge toward the same policy mix (Bennett 1991). The convergence thesis would suggest that end-of-life policies across disparate country environments would have a tendency to become more similar over time as the countries develop economically. Gibson and Means (2000), for example, argue that recent restructuring has led to convergence of the health systems of Australia and the United Kingdom despite quite dissimilar goals and strategic emphases. Based on an examination of trends across industrialized democracies, Chernichovsky (1995) agrees that despite the variety of health care systems, health system reforms have led to the emergence of a universal outline or paradigm for health care financing, organization, and management.

Critics of convergence theories, however, argue that they oversimplify the process of development and underestimate significant divergence across countries (Howlett and Ramish 1995). Convergence, they argue, downplays the importance of country-specific factors other than perhaps economic development, and most studies that find evidence of convergence do not find it applicable across the board, thus allowing for divergence in other areas. This book does not attempt to test the convergence theory, but its current prominence in the literature dictates that its appropriateness to end-of-life policy be addressed in the concluding chapter.

Organization of the Book

This book brings together ethical and policy experts from a range of countries in order to examine how end-of-life policies vary across these countries, what country-specific factors influence these policies, and how terminally ill patients are treated by the respective health care systems. As such, it is hoped this volume will fill a void in the literature, which although it is extensive, contains few works that look at a full range of these issues across more than several nations. Even the broader literature on comparative health policy has tended to include only industrialized, primarily Western, countries, thus giving a skewed picture of the problems and context. As a result, the conceptual debates over various health policy issues, including end-of-life decision making, have become largely framed by Western practices and values. The objective here is to expand the prevailing boundaries of comparative study by including countries that represent a wide range of cultural, economic, and ideological dimensions.

The chapters that follow make it clear that ethical issues as framed in affluent countries dominated by a liberal and capitalist value system cannot easily be extrapolated to countries with less individualistic cultures or lacking the economic resources necessary to achieve such ends. Although there is considerable variation across Western nations (and in some cases within them) regarding end-of-life policies, these differences are even starker in this broader sample of countries.

In order to provide a starting point for discussion and facilitate comparative data, chapter contributors were asked, where possible, to address these questions and issues:

1. What are the estimated costs of dying, per person and in aggregate?

2. What proportion of health care costs is expended in the last 6 months of life? The last 3 months of life?

3. What proportion of the population dies in intensive care units, hospitals, hospices, homes?

4. What proportion dies with some form of advance directive? What forms of advance directives are available? Are they binding?

5. What is the level of availability to pain management?

6. What is the mix of high technology and palliative care?

7. What are cutoff points for aggressive care? Who decides? What is the legal definition of death?

8. What government policies, if any, are operative in end-of-life decisions?

9. What policies, if any, are there for assisted suicide or euthanasia?

10. What agents are most responsible for making these decisions (a government agency, the medical community, ethics committees, the family)?

11. What role does age play, if any, in decisions at the end of life?

12. What factors unique to the country (cultural, social, religious, economic, etc.) are critical for understanding end-of-life decision making in that country?

In the end, the emphasis given to each question varied widely across the chapters, as discussed in more detail in chapter 14. The fact that many authors were unable to uncover even rough data on many of these factors, especially on the first four questions, is itself important in demonstrating the variation in the state of end-of-life policy across these countries.

In order to provide a broad range of studies, the countries in table 1.2 were selected. They represent a good mix of economic, religious, and cultural contexts and are about equally from the West and non-West. They range in population size from 6 million in Israel to more than 1 billion each in India and China. There is also substantial variation along economic lines. While European countries, Japan, and the United States all have a per capita gross domestic product (GDP) of over $20,000, with the United States highest at $33,900, India and Kenya have less than a tenth of that figure at $1,800 and $1,600, respectively. Similarly, while Japan, Taiwan, the Netherlands, and the United States have unemployment rates running under 5 percent, the rate for Kenya is 50 per-

Table 1.2
Countries studied and selected variables

Country	Population (millions)	Gross domestic product per capita (US$)	Unemploy-ment rate (percent)	Population under 15 years (percent)	Population over 65 years (percent)	Life expectancy at birth (years)	Infant mortality (deaths/1,000 births)
Brazil	172	6,150	7.5	29	5	62.9	38.1
China	1,260	3,800	10.0	25	7	71.4	28.9
Germany	83	22,700	10.5	16	16	77.4	4.8
Israel	6	18,300	9.1	28	9	78.6	7.9
India	1,014	1,800	na	34	4	62.5	64.9
Japan	126	23,400	4.7	15	17	80.7	3.9
Kenya	30	1,600	50.0	43	3	48.0	68.7
Netherlands	16	23,100	3.5	18	14	78.3	4.4
Taiwan	22	16,100	2.9	22	8	76.4	7.1
Turkey	66	6,200	7.3	29	6	70.1	49.9
U.K.	59	21,800	6.0	19	16	77.7	5.6
U.S.	275	33,900	4.2	21	13	77.1	6.3

Source: Data from *World Factbook* (2003).
Notes: All numbers are for the year 2000, except GDP and unemployment, which are for 1999. na, not available.

cent. Although these indicators fluctuate from year to year, the relative states of these economies are consistent by country, a factor that is bound to have an impact on the way in which end-of-life decisions are made.

In terms of health, two variables that serve as very rough indicators of the health status of a population are life expectancy at birth and infant mortality rates. Life expectancy is 80.7 years in Japan and over 78 in Israel and the Netherlands. In contrast, life expectancy in Brazil and India is approximately 62 years, and in Kenya it is only 48 years. Likewise, infant mortality rates vary widely, from 3.91 deaths per 1,000 births in Japan to more than 60 per 1,000 births in India and Kenya. Moreover, it might be expected that countries with rapidly aging populations face different pressures than those with relatively young populations. Among our countries again there is wide variation. Countries such as Brazil, Turkey, India, and especially Kenya have extraordinarily high proportions of their populations under age 15, while countries such as Germany, the United Kingdom, and Japan are dealing with large older populations.

Likewise, cultural factors and social values vary across countries, and in some cases are most crucial for end-of-life policy. Values dominant in the West such as individual rights, lifestyle choice, and the dependence on technology to fix all problems, including death, are not universals, despite what much of the bioethics literature assumes (for exceptions, see Alora and Lumitao 2001, and the work of Macer 1998). Moreover, there may be strong cultural and value divisions within a particular country that are important in defining policy. Religious factors are particularly critical dimensions for death-related policies, and in some countries they are the single most important factor. Moreover, social structures can be central to care of the terminally ill and in setting the boundaries of such care. In many countries, extended families and communities still have a central role to play, while in other countries even the nuclear family seems to play a limited role in care giving.

Overall then, the countries represented here offer a wide range of contexts for studying end-of-life policy. We leave it up to the individual authors to describe in more detail the critical cultural, religious, and other factors that affect the end-of-life debate in their respective countries and return briefly in the concluding chapter to discuss the findings as related to the themes and issues.

References

Alora, A. T., and J. M. Lumitao. 2001. *Beyond Western Bioethics: Voices from the Developing World*. Washington, D.C.: Georgetown University Press.

American Academy of Family Physicians. 2003. Definition of Hospice. www.aafp.org/X6864.xml (accessed April 16, 2003).

Bennett, C. J. 1991. "What Is Policy Convergence and What Causes It?" *British Journal of Political Science* 21 (2): 215–233.

Blank, R. H. 1995. *Biomedical Policy*. Chicago: Nelson-Hall.

Chernichovsky, D. 1995. "Health System Reforms in Industrialized Democracies: An Emerging Paradigm." *Milbank Quarterly* 73 (3): 339–356.

Gibson, D., and R. Means. 2000. "Policy Convergence: Restructuring Long-term Care in Australia and the UK." *Policy and Politics* 29 (1): 43–58.

Ham, C. 1997. "Priority Setting in Health Care: Learning From International Experience." *Health Policy* 42 (1): 49–66.

Ham, C. 2001. "Commentary: Values and Health Policy: The Case of Singapore." *Journal of Health Politics, Policy and Law* 26 (4): 746–748.

Harrop, M. 1992. "Health Policy." In *Power and Policy in Liberal Democracies*, edited by Martin Harrop. Cambridge: Cambridge University Press, pp. 1–12.

Howlett, M., and M. Ramesh. 1995. *Studying Public Policy: Policy Cycles and Policy Subsystems*. New York: Oxford University Press.

Immergut, E. M. 1992. *Health Policies: Interests and Institutions in Western Europe*. Cambridge: Cambridge University Press.

Macer, D. 1998. *Bioethics in Asia*. Christchurch, New Zealand: Eubios Ethics Institute. See also the *Eubios Journal of Asian and International Bioethics* (www.biol.tsukuba.ac.jp/~maccr/index.html).

Olick, R. S. 2001. *Taking Advance Directives Seriously: Prospective Autonomy and Decisions Near the End of Life*. Washington, D.C.: Georgetown University Press.

Ovretveit, J. 1998. *Comparative and Cross-Cultural Health Research*. Abingdon, UK: Radcliffe Medical Press.

Sass, H.-M., R. M. Veatch, and R. Kimura, eds. 1998. *Advance Directives and Surrogate Decision Making in Health Care: United States, Germany, and Japan*. Baltimore, Md.: Johns Hopkins University Press.

Webb, M., T. E. Quill, and J. Lynn. 1997. *The Good Death: The New American Search to Reshape the End of Life*. New York: Doubleday Dell.

Weir, R. F. 1989. *Abating Treatment with Critically Ill Patients*. New York: Oxford University Press.

Wijdicks, E. F. M., ed. 2001. *Brain Death*. New York: Lippincott Williams and Wilkins.

World Factbook. 2003. http://education.yahoo.com/reference/factbook (accessed June 6, 2003).

World Health Organization. 2002. www5.who.int (accessed October 4).

2

Ethical Questions Related to End-of-Life Decisions: The Brazilian Reality

Léo Pessini

It is a challenge to reflect on ethical grounds about the dying process, for in Brazil to date there has been little discussion of these ethical issues. This chapter begins with an analysis of futile treatment in the codified Brazilian medical ethical tradition. It also examines emerging Brazilian legislation linked to the ethics of end-of-life decisions in São Paulo State and presents some ethical reflections by Brazilian doctors. I also discuss Brazilian legislation on organ donations and transplants, assistance aimed at reducing pain and suffering in the context of the Brazilian health system, and the implementation of the first programs for palliative care in Brazil.

Absolute Respect for Life and the Duty of Not Extending Therapy

One of the remarkable aspects of codified medical ethics in Brazil is its secular as opposed to religious character; it is imbued by humanitarian values and founded on humanist and philosophical concerns. In this context, death and the accompanying suffering are frequently perceived as something without sense, and as they begin to escape from the doctor's control, he tends to see their existence as a failure on his part. The emphasis is on providing the maximum possible length of life, with less concern for the quality of this prolonged life. The consequence is resistance to passive euthanasia, which is understood as a victory for the enemy that is death.

Brazilian medicine uses the following codes: (1) Code of Medical Ethics, adapted from the Code of Medical Ethics of the American

Medical Association in 1867; (2) Code of Medical Morality—1929; (3) Code of Medical Deontology—1931; (4) Code of Medical Deontology—1945; (5) Code of Ethics of Brazilian Medical Association—1953; (6) Code of Medical Ethics—1965; (7) Brazilian Code of Medical Deontology—1984; and the last one, still in force, (8) Code of Medical Ethics—1988 (Martin 1993).[1]

The first code of medical ethics to be adopted in Brazil in 1867 was a Brazilian translation and adaptation of the Code of Medical Ethics of the American Medical Association. It is remarkable the way the profile of the doctor is presented in explicitly religious language:

Article 1—§4 In order to be a minister of hope and solace to his patients, the doctor must encourage the collapsing spirit, soften the bed of death, reanimate the life that is terminating, and be careful of the depressive influence of those illnesses that many times disturb the peace of the most resigned in their last moments. The sick person's life can be shortened not only by the actions but also by the words or manners of the doctor. It is thus a sacred duty to proceed with all care as regards death, avoiding everything that could discourage the sick person or depress his spirit.
§5 The doctor must not abandon the sick person because of judging the disease incurable; his assistance could continue to be very useful to the sick person, as well as giving comfort to the families, even in the last stage of an unfortunate disease. The doctor must alleviate the sick person's suffering and calm his agony of spirit. (Martin 1993: 305–306)

In this profile (demonstrated by the expressions "minister of hope and solace," "encouraging the collapsing spirit," "sacred duty," "calm his agony of spirit") the doctor acts as a clergyman. The code comes from the second part of the nineteenth century, when medicine had few technological means to effectively intervene in the defense of life; thus there is no talk of combating death or of prolonging life. This picture undergoes a complete change in the middle of the twentieth century with the introduction of intensive-care procedures to protect life. From then on, there is a declaration of war on disease and death.

In Brazil, the tradition of codified medical ethics tends to support aggressive intervention. For instance, one of the first Brazilian codes of medical ethics, the code of 1931, discourages the use of euthanasia "because one of the most sublime purposes of Medicine is always [to] maintain and prolong life" (Article 16/31). If we accept that the goal of medicine is always to maintain and prolong life, and the subsequent Brazilian codes follow this direction, we are clearly providing a basis for justifying what might be futile efforts using therapeutic procedures that interfere with the terminal patient's ability to die in peace.

In the code in force since 1988, there was another change of emphasis. The goal of medicine now is not only to provide the maximum period of life but also to maximize the person's health. The criterion for evaluating life-prolongation procedures is their possible benefit for the sick person (Article 2). The commitment to health, where health is understood as the overall well-being of the person rather than the mere absence of disease, makes possible other considerations for the treatment of the terminal patient besides those linked to cure. However, there continues to exist the strong conviction from the earlier codes that the "doctor must have an absolute respect for human life" (Article 6).

This conflict between benefiting the patient with palliative measures that could shorten his or her life but that promote physical and mental well-being on one hand, and the absoluteness of the value of human life in its biological sense, on the other, generates a dilemma that some doctors prefer to solve in favor of prolonging life. With the 1984 and 1988 codes there begins a new approach in which terminal patients have the right not to have treatment extended, to have pain alleviated, but not to have life taken by the doctor. This new phase was due to the emergence of new factors, primarily the progress of medical science.

The 1984 code has perceptible tensions inherent in an alliance of humanitarian benignity with the scientific-technological model as well as with an authoritarian doctor centrism. The humanitarian benignity insists on the "absolute respect for life," already a requirement of the codes of 1953 and 1965 and reinforced by principle 9 in the 1984 code by adding the sentence "from conception to death." The problems this entails center on the fact that this validation of life normally translates as a concern for the maximum prolongation of biological life with an attendant disregard for the quality of the life prolonged. As Leonard Martin states:

[W]ith the emphasis on the biological, suffering, pain and death itself begin to be seen more as technical problems to be solved than experiences lived by persons. The price paid for the good functioning of technology is the depersonalization of pain and death in the Intensive-Care Units, with all their impressive machinery. One can prolong life, but these successful interventions allow for new questions: when is it possible to stop using artificial life-sustaining means? When does death really occur? Is it possible to talk about active and passive euthanasia? (Martin 1993: 216)

There appears to be a tendency to validate a natural death in Article 6 of the 1988 code when it states that it is unethical for the doctor to use "his knowledge to create physical or moral suffering." But what is more significant is Article 61, which encourages doctors to not abandon the patient because he has "a chronic or incurable disease" and to give him "support, if only to mitigate the physical or psychic suffering." This concern to mitigate not only physical but also psychological suffering is a reflection of a new attitude that transcends the mere biological level of physical pain and manifests a concern for the well-being of the person as a whole.

This new attitude is reflected in the recognition of the patient's right to not have treatment extended. In the codes of 1984 (Article 23) and 1988 (Article 69), there is a prohibition against extending treatment. "The intentional complication of the patient's treatment, by means of either medicines having uncertain results or by way of nonconventional surgical practices used with the only aim of experimenting with a new technique or venture in more bold alternatives" must be avoided according to França (1997: 65). In his comments on Article 56 of the 1988 code of medical ethics, Franca states that "the doctor is not allowed to disregard the patient's right to freely decide on the use of diagnostic or therapeutic practices, except in cases of impending death" (França 1997: 62).

The concept of medical futility begins to gain more space in the discussions about bioethics, mainly in cases of prolongation of life for seriously ill patients as well as in conditions considered irreversible. Now-a-days it is possible to view as futile treatments those treatments that do not benefit the patient, that are useless or inefficacious, that do not offer a minimum quality of life and where there is no possibility of survival. (Franca 1997: 62)

Another important aspect of the 1988 code regarding the patient's right not to have treatment extended is concern for regulating medical research that treats terminal patients as subjects. Article 130 prohibits the doctor from experimenting "with new clinical or surgical treatments using patients with non-curable or terminal diseases when there is no reasonable hope of benefiting the patient, avoiding inflicting on him additional suffering" (Conselho Federal de Medicina 1988: 1577). While the code recognizes the legitimacy of recourse to experimental treatments, it establishes a well-defined criterion: the existence of a "reasonable hope" that the treatment will be beneficial for the sick person and the certainty that no avoidable sufferings will be inflicted on him.

Emerging Brazilian Legislation: São Paulo State

On March 17, 1999, São Paulo State promulgated Act 10.241, which "makes provisions for the rights of users of health services and actions in the State and for other purposes." The act had as its origin Proposition 546/97 of Representative Roberto Gouveia (Brazilian Workers' Party), who was inspired by the booklet of patients' rights published in 1995 by the Conselho Estadual de Saúde (State Council for Health Matters). The booklet was based on a proposal elaborated by Fórum de Patologias do Estado de São Paulo (São Paulo State's Pathologies Forum), a strong nongovernmental organization, with the collaboration of the Pastoral Care of the National Conference of Brazilian Bishops (Gouveia 2000).

Act 10.241 has two articles and two appendices. Elaborated in humanist terms, it is concerned with giving the patient a central place regarding health-care questions and avoiding the increasing dehumanization of health institutions where a sick person is considered a passive object of health care. Appendix XXIII refers especially to the terminal patient or one for whom there are no therapeutic possibilities, in the language of palliative medicine specialists. The act grants to the user or his or her legal representative the right to refuse painful or extraordinary treatments aiming to prolong life. Appendix XXIV refers to the choice of the place where one will die:

Article 2. The users of health services of São Paulo State are entitled to the following rights:
XXIII—to refuse painful or out of the ordinary treatments aiming to prolong life; and
XXIV—to choose the place where to die. (Gouveia 2000: 180)

Due respect for the sick person implies not forcing on him or her, through paternalistic beneficence, something the patient does not want, even as she or he approaches death. There must be respect for the patient's self-determination and autonomy. Every person has the right to choose to die with quality of life at the place he or she prefers and it is the doctor's duty to always act in the patient's best interests.

Article 57 of the Brazilian Code of Medical Ethics of 1988 states "in no way can a doctor not employ every available diagnostic and treatment measures to benefit the patient." Notwithstanding these provisions, says Gabriel Oselka, the former president of the Brazilian Federal Council of Medicine, many doctors misunderstand the article and inter pret it as saying that they are forced to do everything in every situation, even when there is no way to prevent death. Besides, they fear being accused of omitting assistance, something that is a crime under the Brazilian Penal Code of 1940, which is being revised. Brazilian intensive care units are a clear example of the dilemma:

[A] great many patients are kept artificially alive by means of machinery and medicines; they do not really prolong life, but only postpone death, frequently causing suffering. No doubt many patients would prefer that extraordinary procedures be stopped if they were told their clinical condition is irreversible. In terminal cases, it would be more beneficial and respectful for the patient that instead of using out of the ordinary procedures, the professionals alleviate pain and give comfort, letting nature follow its normal course and the patient cease to exist in peace. (Lemes 2000: 127)

It is important to emphasize that this is not abandonment or omission of assistance, much less euthanasia.

Along in the same line, in his comment on appendices XXIII and XXIV of Act 10.241, the moral theologian Márcio Fabri dos Anjos concludes:

[L]ife's unnecessary prolongation at all costs when death is unavoidable is dysthanasia (from Greek *dis* + *thanasia*), "slow death," an anxious and much painful death. Dysthanasia can even be considered violence, as it subjects the person to painful or degrading therapeutic procedures without any sense. Thus, incise XXIII contributes to humanizing terminality. (Lemes 2000: 128)

Since the patient now has the right to choose the place to die, this opens an interesting possibility for developing home-care procedures and for introducing the philosophy of palliative home care in the Brazilian health system.[2]

Ethical Considerations on the Codes of Medical Ethics and Dysthanasia

Dysthanasia and euthanasia have in common the aspect of causing death "in the wrong hour." With dysthanasia it is not possible to determine when therapeutic interventions are useless or when it is advisable to accept that people should die in peace as the natural outcome of life. The one value this procedure seeks to protect is human life. Whereas euthanasia is based on a concern for the *quality* of the remaining life, dysthanasia tends to focus on the *quantity* of life and aims to use all possible measures to extend the life span to the maximum (Martin 1998).

It is argued here that a better understanding of the practice of dysthanasia could be obtained by situating it in the transition of medicine as an art—in its premodern expressions—to medicine as a technique and as a science—in its more contemporary expressions. Technological and scientific advances, as well as the success attained in treating a great many human diseases, has forced medicine to concentrate on the cure of pathologies and move to the background the more traditional concern of caring for the sick person. In this perspective, the technical question is how to prolong the vital signs of a severely ill person; terminality is determined by objective criteria such as progressive and multiple organ failures. The difficult ethical question that arises is what sense all this makes and what should be the limits in pursuing this course.

Another important challenge is how to define when death really occurs. Today, the accepted criterion in Brazil is that of cerebral, or brain, death. Although in most cases there is no doubt about the patient's death and both the medical team and the family accept it without questioning, other cases are not so clear. The increasing acceptance of brain death for determining human death in Brazil is a decisive factor not only for allowing the family to make funeral arrangements but also for using body organs in transplants (Lepargneur 1993).

The distinction between therapy and basic care opens possibilities for ethical measures that avoid futile treatment. Care for the patient's hygiene, well-being, and oral nutrition are no doubt normal care measures. The ethical obligation to use every other means of medical or therapeutic procedures, including artificial nutrition, must be evaluated by taking into consideration the relation between the burden imposed on the patients and those who care for them, and the benefits that can reasonably be expected. There is no obligation to begin and continue medical intervention when the suffering or efforts required are not proportional to the expected benefits. In these cases, what causes death is not the interruption of therapy, but rather the preexisting pathological process.

However tentative, the discussion about futile treatment in Brazilian medicine is beginning to show some positive signs, as demonstrated by the efforts of intensive care experts, who are sensitive to the issues involved. They have refused to import solutions from abroad (mainly from the United States), instead insisting on making decisions based on Brazilian cultural heritage.[3] Taking into account Brazilian culture, Délio Kipper points to three issues:

> [W]e question ourselves as concerns our decisions about the end of life; (a) because we have the clear perception that we still use technology excessively and inappropriately, senselessly prolonging human suffering, making a bad use of scarce financial resources destined to health-care and needlessly using the always limited number of beds in ICUs and emergency rooms; (b) from a legal standpoint, we feel we have no legal provisions that help us to decide on not offering or interrupting vital sustaining measures; (c) we feel a lack of regulations and rules on how to treat these [terminal] patients. (Kipper 1999: 66)

Kipper offers the following proposal for item (a) of his comments. As soon as brain death is confirmed according to Resolution 1480/97 (Conselho Federal de Medicina 1997),[4] doctors must inform the family and explain the inability of medicine to reverse the patient's condition, allowing them time to reflect on and comprehend the situation, before stopping the use of artificial means for maintaining vegetative functions. The interval between the occurrence of brain death and notification of the family must not be more than 24 hours lest it be considered therapeutic obstinacy. Kipper adds that doctors must provide for the well-being of terminal patients through palliative measures and support for the family. He favors withholding cardiopulmonary resuscitation in accord with the will of the patient and/or the family and avoiding treatments deemed futile or disproportionate.

In regard to legislation (item b), Kipper sees as imperative a revision of the Brazilian Penal Code that includes a clause that exempts the physician from responsibility in these cases. In addition, there are provisions for decriminalizing the termination of support systems when two doctors have verified that death is impending and unavoidable and the patient or a legal representative has given their consent. To date, however, there is no specific regulation that protects a doctor's decision to withhold or discontinue resuscitation efforts; thus it remains a legal risk for the health professional (Abdala 1997). Given the absence of regulations and rules, it is no longer possible to postpone a broad discussion involving society to determine what provisions can be proposed for guiding doctors, patients, and families. An example of a regulatory proposal is Report 12/98 (Conselho Federal de Medicina 1988), which recognizes the criterion of brain death for all patients, irrespective of organ donors.

The Brazilian Penal Code has been under revision since the early 1980s. As of January 9, 2002, there was a first draft that changes the code's provisions affecting euthanasia. In the Special Section, Article 121, Title I, number 3, on crimes against the individual, the code states: "If the author of the crime acted by compassion, at the request of the victim, being legally imputable and beyond the age of majority, with an aim to shorten unbearable physical suffering due to a severe disease, the penalty is three to six years of prison." What has a direct link to our discussion is number 4, which decriminalizes the refusal to maintain life artificially when there is no hope of survival:

It is not considered a crime the action to stop artificial maintenance of life when death has been attested to by two doctors as impending and unavoidable and when there is consent of the patient or, when the patient cannot decide, of an ascendant, descendant, spouse or sibling.

According to Kipper, the context of medical decisions on the ending of life is always unique, critical, and entirely individual both for the doctor and for the patient and the family. There are fewer complications when there is a good doctor-patient-family relationship and there is the conviction that the proposed procedure is the best one for the specific patient, in the specific place, and at the specific time.

Dialogue is the key term in the relationship of doctor, patient, and family. According to Mota (1999), professionals who work with critically ill patients need intensive and extensive training in techniques for the preservation and/or restoration of vital functions. In addition, they ought to be prepared to reflect on all the related questions and to engage in a dialogue with all involved parties, having as interlocutors patients, the family, and other professionals related to the patient's care. This dialogue must have as its goal the best interest of the patient. At the same time, it has to take into account the fact that science alone cannot answer ethical questions, although it is able to contribute by means of data analysis and scientific perspectives. At their core, the choices always stem from ethical decisions. This is the ethical challenge present in the care of critically ill patients: when and how to act, doing the best to promote their interests without crossing the line to futile measures. This is a difficult task, requiring considerably more than the mere knowledge of life-sustaining technologies.

Following this humanist track, Horta sums up very well what is involved in this question:

When physical life is considered a supreme and absolute value, beyond liberty and dignity, excessive love for life becomes idolatry. Medicine promotes implicitly this blind worship of life, organizing the terminal stage of life as combating death at all costs. It is our urgent task to rebel against this ideological view of dying. Brazilian medicine and society have before them an ethical challenge that they must urgently meet: humanize life in its decline, giving it back its lost dignity. Hundreds or maybe thousands of sick persons are now forced to suffer without hope in hospitals, mainly in intensive-care units and emergency rooms. Most of them are subjected to a technological panoply that not only is incapable of alleviating their pain and suffering but uselessly prolongs and increases them. (Horta 1993: 228)

It is important to note the point of view of José Eduardo Siqueira, eminent Brazilian cardiologist and vice-president of the Sociedade Brasileira de Bioética (Brazilian Bioethics Society). In his comments on employing technology in intensive care units, he says:

In fact, our intensive-care units began to care as well for incurable chronic patients with many associated diseases who now have the same status as severely ill ones. While for the latter a full restoration is frequently attainable, for the chronically ill patients one offers little more than a precarious survival and many times merely vegetative existence. This is the situation known as therapeutic obstinacy, futility in Anglophone [English-speaking] countries and "encarnizamiento" [cruelty] in Hispanic ones. How far must we go in our use of technological procedures for sustaining life? The Cartesian model of medicine teaches us a lot about cutting-edge technology but little about the metaphysical meaning of life and death. ... The education we received taught us to understand life as a strictly biological phenomenon, and we assimilated biomedical technology to pursue this utopia. The obsession with maintaining biological life at all costs guided us to therapeutic obstinacy. Thus, we have before us a most relevant ethical dilemma: when must we not use available technology? (Siqueira 2000: 62–63)

São Paulo State's Conselho Regional de Medicina (Regional Council of Medicine) recently published the book *Aids e Ética Médica* (Aids and Medical Ethics). The work presents an interesting sample of the way doctors see the ethical decision process regarding the ending of life. In the entry on euthanasia, which actually speaks about futile treatment, there are some initial comments about Brazilian legislation and the current code of medical ethics documents that prohibit euthanasia (Article 66). The text in full reads:

The degree to which the doctor has the obligation to try to prolong the life of a terminal patient, the type of resources he is forced to use in these circumstances and the right of the patient to give his opinion about the matter merit discussion. Passive medical euthanasia, or euthanasia by omission, corresponds to the non-utilization of means aimed at prolonging the life of incurable patients, something that allows for the natural evolution of death. There is now a broad acceptance that the doctor has no legal, moral, or ethical obligation to use, in irreversible cases, measures that serve only to make the process of dying longer.

It is nevertheless evident that some situations are possible where the doctor is undecided about what course to follow. To help him or her, it is important to discuss the therapeutic options and their implications. Although it is only a guiding principle for the doctor's decision, the patient's (or the family's) will is obviously a welcome aid. To facilitate this, living wills are becoming increasingly common (Conselho Regional de Medicina do Estado de São Paulo 2001). This indicates a new direction in end-of-life questions. Fortunately, there are now encouraging signs of this change of perspective, a perspective that goes beyond technological capabilities and considers the entire human being.

Brazilian Legislation on Organ Transplants

The first act (5479) on the use of tissues, organs, and parts of dead bodies for therapeutic and scientific ends was passed in August 1968, several months after the first heart transplant in Brazil (May 26, 1968) was performed at the Hospital das Clínicas (General Hospital) of the

Faculdade de Medicina da Universidade de São Paulo (Medical School of University of São Paulo). In February 1997, Act 9434 went into effect and implementation of a national policy and a national system for transplants began. This is the positive side of the regulation. The increase in the number of transplants in the past 2 years was over 50 percent, making Brazil the second country in terms of absolute number of transplants, ranking behind only the United States.

However, many patients die before they receive a transplant because while transplant services have been able to increase the number of surgeries, not enough organs are available. Some 25 percent of the families with a member who is declared brain dead refuse to donate organs. In Brazil, there are only 4 donors per 1 million persons each year. This is only one-tenth the rate in the more developed countries. This translates into a great challenge in terms of education concerning this issue. Added to this is the frequent specter of the commercialization of organs. Although denounced widely, there is no proof of this and no one has ever gone to prison for engaging in such practices, although it has recently been reported that poor Brazilians had traveled to South Africa, where they were paid approximately $10,000 per kidney (Desperation 2004). Table 2.1 presents data from the Central of Transplantes of São Paulo State (Transplant Center) and the Associação Brasileira de Transplantes

Table 2.1
Transplants in Brazil and São Paulo State and waiting recipients in São Paulo, 2001

	Transplants		Waiting recipients,
Organ/tissue	Brazil 2003	São Paulo 2001	São Paulo 2001
Cornea	6286	2484	4091
Kidney	3126	553	9932
Liver	792	242	1881
Heart	175	65	65
Pancreas/kidney	163	54	178
Pancreas	50	26	51
Lungs	38	4	10

Sources: Central of Transplantes of São Paulo State; Associação Brasileira de Transplantes.

(Brazilian Transplant Association) on the number of transplants in Brazil and São Paulo and the number of persons awaiting a transplant in São Paulo.

In 1997, health officials and technocrats tried to impose presumed donation of organs, that is, the concept that everyone is a donor unless they have a document expressly refusing to do so. However, there was a spontaneous mass protest against presumed donation; 97 percent of the population declared themselves nondonors in documents such as their identification card and driver's license. The regulation almost undermined the credibility and viability of the Brazilian transplant system and it became necessary to change the law. This protest caused the alteration of Act 9434 by a new provision (MP 1718, October 6, 1998) that states: "If a potential donor does not manifest his will, a father, mother, descendant or spouse can manifest his refusal as concerns organ donation, and this manifestation is mandatory for the transplant and donation teams." A further regulation (MP 1959–27, October 20, 2000) states: "The manifestations of will as regards post mortem disposal of tissues, organs and dead body parts included in Carteira de Identidade civil [ID card] and Carteira Nacional de Habilitação [national driver's license] will be no longer in force from March 1, 2001."

On March 23, 2001, a new transplant law (10.211) was enacted that formally annulled presumed donation and gave the family the power to give permission for transplants. Thus, 3 years later, the annullment of the mandatory organ donation act reflected a Brazilian cultural, moral, and social reality that favors the principle of liberty and autonomy to decide what to do with one's body.

Alleviation of Pain and Suffering in the Final Stages of Life

In considering health care in Brazil, it is important to approach the question of alleviating pain and suffering in the final stages of life in the broader context of Brazilian culture, marked as it is by an amazing passivity in attitudes toward pain, within a social milieu in which inequalities and exclusion prevail, a legacy of our past of slavery and religious indoctrination ("the poor must suffer" and the faithful no less, in order to "go to heaven").

In Brazil at the federal government level there is now a national program of permanent education in pain and palliative care for health professionals.[5] The International Association for the Study of Pain defines pain in scientific terms as "An unpleasant sensory and emotional experience associated with actual or potential tissue damage, or described in terms of such damage" (Figueiró 2000: 67). Pain is generally ignored by health professionals and educators responsible for designing the curricula of the field's professionals.[6] There are few epidemiological studies that focus on the frequency and distribution of pain in the population, and the topic is still little discussed in Brazil. However, there is evidence that pain is the main cause of 75 to 80 percent of visits to the primary health care system. Chronic pain affects a great many persons in Brazil, and it is considered the main cause of absenteeism at work, sick leave, low productivity, early retirements, and indemnities for workers. In Brazil, six of the eleven most purchased pharmaceuticals in 1998 were analgesics and anti-inflammatories (Figueiró 2000).

Pain is still a long way from receiving due consideration in Brazilian health assistance systems. Educational programs about pain for patients, doctors, pharmacists, nurses, psychologists, social workers, and other professionals are needed. The challenge for the scientific community, health professionals, and society as a whole is to establish a special program for training these professionals in pain alleviation. It is imperative to discuss and give explanations about pain in order to promote a better understanding of pain and better preventive measures as well as its control (see Centro Universitário São Camilo 1988; see also Pimenta et al. 1997).

Traditionally, the medical schools organized their undergraduate curriculum according to the Flexner Report on Medical Education, written in 1912, a text based on a biological, technology-centered vision of clinical teaching. Thus the human body was studied in a fragmented way, and disease was considered a malfunction of biological mechanisms studied according to the perspective of molecular and cellular biology. Medical procedures intervened physically or chemically in order to normalize the functioning of the affected unit. The objective of medical schools was to train experts in disease, not physicians dedicated to caring for sick people. Modern concerns about the relationship among psychological, social, and cultural conditions, however, have indicated the need to include an integrated, holistic concept of the patient in basic clinical training. This change in focus must be reflected in academic curricula that train medical personnel to address all the needs of patients—to promote their physical, psychic, and social well-being (Carvalho 1999).[7]

There are now initial efforts in health institutions for health care based on a palliative care philosophy. The Associação Brasileira de Cuidados Paliativos (Brazilian Association for Palliative Care), founded in São Paulo State in 1997, offers great hope for the practical introduction in Brazil of a palliative care philosophy. Among the reasons for the foundation of this association are:

Palliative medicine is acquiring an increasing relevance in the entire world, assimilating the concept of caring instead of only curing. The patient begins to be considered as a being that suffers physically, psychologically, socially and spiritually. Palliative-care measures aim to control pain, alleviate symptoms and improve quality of life in accordance with a multidisciplinary approach. (Associação Brasileira de Cuidados Paliativos 1998: 191).

The association has among its aims (1) promoting scientific and professional integration for professionals that study and practice disciplines linked to care regarding chronic diseases, diseases in advanced stages, and terminal illnesses; (2) improving the quality of attention given to sick persons affected by chronic pathologies; (3) encouraging research in palliative care by means of congresses, seminars, and conferences, aiming to improve the professional, technical, and scientific knowledge of all health professionals; (4) developing, advising and giving technical assistance in matters related to the content and curriculum of academic programs of training in the health field; (5) promoting studies and discussions on ethical issues and their implications for palliative care procedures; and (6) promoting the well-being of the community and preserving an improved quality of life for sick people at several health-care levels.

A report by this association reveals that as of 1998 there were only twenty-nine palliative care centers in Brazil for ambulatory patients and patients admitted to hospitals, as well as those at home. Almost all of them are extensions of pain-alleviation services. Among the current challenges, the association notes: (1) the absence of a national policy on pain alleviation; (2) deficiencies in both the training of health professionals and the education of the community; (3) concerns about the abuse of morphine and other opium derivatives, something that causes increasing restrictions on morphine prescriptions and the drug's availability; (4) restrictions on supplying and distributing other drugs necessary to alleviate pain and other symptoms; (5) deficiencies in the training of health professionals responsible for the prescription of analgesics and other drugs; and (6) lack of financial resources for research and development in the field of palliative care (Pessini and Bertachini, 2004).

There are at this initial stage encouraging signs in Brazilian medicine regarding the introduction of palliative care, if not concrete measures, at least in the form of a concern. Some academic works—master's dissertations, doctoral theses, and many seminars and events—are appearing that have palliative care as their focus. For example, in her doctoral thesis Maria Guerra focused on the care of AIDS patients according to a palliative care philosophy. The ideal to be attained is to:

develop a general consciousness as regards the importance to care, mainly when curing is no longer a possibility; of the relevances of the concept of total pain, with its physical, psychic and spiritual components; of respect for the sick person's concerns; of the acceptance of death as an event as natural as birth, an event health professionals must assist, by guiding, preventing complications, alleviating the accompanying suffering, helping to make it a less hurtful event, an event that dignifies all people involved. (Guerra 2001: 136)

Brazilian medicine has some professionals who are outspoken defenders of a practice that cares for human beings as spiritually as well as physically. Eminent Brazilian physicians frequently make their voices heard in national newspapers, reflecting on ethical questions that medicine has to answer at the end of life. One of these is Miguel Srougi, from Escola Paulista de Medicina (São Paulo State Medical School). In his comments on the deaths of Governor Mário Covas and Doctor Cutait, a famous São Paulo State physician, he states:

When we take into account the fears that terminal patients are haunted by, we conclude that physicians will only be able to play their role completely if they assume the position they had in remote times when, guided by spiritual and religious values, they were the guardians of both body and soul. Another condition for this is to mix their efficient elixirs that alleviate physical suffering with three magic potions whose effects are almost sublime: listen without judging, express themselves from a superior dimension, and be always present. (Srougi 2001: A–3)

A cursory reading of this professional attitude could see it as a romantic longing for medical practice as a kind of priestly role, something prevalent in earlier times in Brazil, but not possible in today's health care market–technology-driven reality.

Concluding Remarks

This overview of ethical questions related to end-of-life medical decisions began with a discussion of codified Brazilian medical ethics and then analyzed the Brazilian pioneering legislation, Act 10.241 (March 17, 1999) of São Paulo State and the Brazilian codes of medical ethics. It is clear that Brazilian medicine is now in a paradigm shift. Because legislation tends to have as its basis a certain model of medicine, as this model undergoes change, legislation and ethical codes also change. Regarding the dying process, this change can occur only by an intervention in the very core of the system: health professionals, especially physicians, must learn to view their practice from a more humane and ethically founded perspective, a point of view that goes beyond the unilateral idolizing of excellence in terms of mere technological competence.

In Brazil, ethical-medical questions linked to end-of-life decisions are still surrounded by a curtain of silence. There are limited statistical data on death. This silence has gradually begun to be broken by efforts to reformulate medical school curricula as well as by an increasing number of conferences and other events that discuss and seek to better understand the questions involved from a bioethical perspective. The ever-increasing expansion of bioethics in Brazil shows that changes are under way. There is now a great hope that health care in Brazil will have a more humane face, a face that respects human dignity. There are signs of an increasing concern to humanize health services, especially intensive care units, as well as to implement a palliative care philosophy. Some pioneering projects exist that try to base terminal patient care on this philosophy.

Notes

1. Martin (1993) appendices contain the full text of all codes of medical ethics used in Brazil.

2. São Paulo State's main newspapers gave great prominence to this new state provision. In *Folha de São Paulo* March 20, 1999, for instance, we read: Lei Permite a Recusa de Procedimentos Dolorosos e a Escolha do Local da Morte

(Act Allows for Refusal of Painful Procedures and Choice of Place to Die). In gigantic letters, the headline states Paciente Ganha o Direito Legal de Recusar Tratamento (Patient is Given Legal Rights to Refuse Treatment). The featured article quotes many experts in medicine and other fields, e.g., bioethics and religion, and shows that a consensus exists (Russo 1999). For the president of the Sociedade Brasileira de Bioética (Brazilian Bioethics Society), Prof. Marcos Segre, the legislation "consolidates the consensus according to which patients must not obey doctors, assigning the patient the role of an agent."

3. Brazil's Federal Council of Medicine has for 11 years now published the journal *Bioética* (Bioethics). It is a pioneering effort, and its editorial line promotes the interdisciplinary and pluralistic discussion of the questions involved. I was personally responsible, together with Júlio Cesar Meirelles Gomes, M.D., for coordinating a symposium on euthanasia for the first issue (1999).

4. Resolution 1480/97 establishes criteria for determining the total and irreversible failure of encephalic functions in persons aged 2 years or older.

5. Compare the report that presents arguments for the need to provide this governmental program at the Brazilian federal level in Centro Universitário São Camilo (1988).

6. There are basically two kinds of pain: acute pain and chronic pain. Acute pain is in general associated with some kind of body wound and tends to disappear when the wound heals. Chronic pain is pain that goes on for more than 6 months.

7. This is a reference work in the medical field on caring for pain and suffering. Most of the contributions are multidisciplinary.

References

Abdalla, L. A. 1997. Aspectos éticos e médico-legais da ressuscitação cardiopulmonar-ordens de não ressuscitar. *Revista da Sociedade de Cardiologia do Estado de São Paulo* 7 (1): 175–181.

Associação Brasileira de Cuidados Paliativos. 1998. Informe. *O Mundo da Saúde,* May/June, p. 191.

Carvalho, M. J. de (Org.). 1999. *Dor: um Estudo Multidisciplinar.* São Paulo: Summus Editorial.

Centro Universitário São Camilo. 1988. *O Mundo da Saúde,* January-February.

Conselho Federal de Medicina. 1988. Código de Ética Médica—resolução CFM n. 1246/88. In *Diário Oficial da União,* January, 26 1988. Section 1, 1574–77. Brasília: Imprensa Nacional.

Conselho Federal de Medicina. 1999. *Bioética* 1 (1).

Conselho Federal de Medicina. *Resolução 1997. CFM* number 1480. http://www.cfm.org.br/97.htm. (accessed November 29, 2000).

Conselho Regional de Medicina do Estado de São Paulo. 2001. *Aids e Ética Médica.* São Paulo: Conselho Regional de Medicina do Estado de São Paulo.

"Desperation and Sympathy Impel the Illegal Purchase of a Kidney." *International Herald Tribune*, May 24, 2004.

Figueiró, J. A. 2000. *A dor*. São Paulo: Publifolha.

França, G. V. De. 1987. *Medicina Legal*, 2nd ed. Rio de Janeiro: Guanabara Koogan.

França, G. V. De. 1993. *Comentários ao Código de Ética Médica*. Rio de Janeiro: Guanabara Koogan.

Gouveia, R. 2000. *Saúde Pública, Suprema Lei: A Nova Legislação para a Conquista da Saúde*. São Paulo: Mandacaru.

Guerra, M. A. T. 2001. Assistência ao paciente em fase terminal: alternativa para o doente com AIDS. Ph.D. thesis, Departamento de Práticas de Saúde da Faculdade de Saúde Pública, Universidade de São Paulo.

Horta, M. P. 1993. Paciente crônico—paciente terminal—eutanásia—problemas éticos da morte e do morrer. In Conselho Federal de Medicina. *Desafios Éticos*. Brasília: Conselho Federal de Medicina, p. 228.

Kipper, D. 1999. O problema das decisões médicas envolvendo o fim da vida e propostas para nossa realidade. *Bioética* 7 (1): 59–70.

Lemes, C. 2000. Direitos tornam-se lei. In R. Gouveia, *Saúde Pública, Suprema Lei: a Nova Legislação Para a Conquista da Saúde*. São Paulo: Mandacaru.

Lepargneur, H. 1993. Morte cerebral. *Revista Eclesiástica Brasileira* 209: 87–98.

Martin, L. M. 1993. *A ética médica diante do paciente terminal: leitura ético teológica da relação médico-paciente terminal nos códigos brasileiros de ética médica*. Aparecida: Santuário.

Martin, L. M. 1998. Eutanásia e distanásia. In Costa, S. I. F., G. Oselka and V. Bottle, eds., *Iniciação à Bioética*. Brasília: Conselho Federal de Medicina, pp. 171–192.

Mello, A. G. Cavalcanti de, Cuidados paliativos: uma abordagem no Brasil. *Boletim informativo do Instituto Camiliano de Pastoral da Saúde*, 189: 3–4, 2001.

Mota, J. C. 1999. Quando um tratamento torna-se fútil? *Bioética* 7 (1): 35–39.

Pessini, L., and L. Bertachini, eds. 2004. *Humanicão e Cuidados Paliativos*. São Paulo: Edições Loyola and Centro Universitário São Camilo.

Pimenta C. A., M. S. Koizumi, and M. J. Teixeira 1997. Dor no doente com câncer: característica e controle. *Revista Brasileira de Cancerologia* 43 (1): 21–44. http://www.inca.org.br/rbc/n_43/v01/artigo2_completo.html (accessed April 20, 2002).

Russo, N. 1999. Lei permite a recusa de procedimentos dolorosos e a escolha do local da morte. *Folha de São Paulo*, March 20, p. 57.

Siqueira, J. E. de. 2000. Tecnologia e medicina entre encontros e desencontros. *Bioética* 8 (1): 55–64.

Srougi, M. 2001. Covas, cutait e o morrer. *Folha de São Paulo*, June 2, p. A–3.

3

End-of-Life Care in China: A View from Beijing

Li Yiting, Ole Döring, Liu Fang, Fu Li, and Su Baoqi

This chapter offers an overview of cultural, social, ethical, and moral dimensions in end-of-life care in contemporary China. It is a pilot study in the sense that it explores the present situation in the emerging sector of hospices and other units for end-of-life care, providing a first account of the situation based upon the professional experiences of a group of experts at Beijing's Capital University of Medical Sciences. It lays out the social and cultural background in China for the particular problems surrounding decision making at the end of life.

In China, death and the dying process are largely matters of professional and private decisions inside the family or in hospitals. This makes it difficult for researchers to obtain and analyze the relevant data. As yet, there is no comprehensive study on the overall situation. Even studies with a narrow regional scope, like this one, have to rely on a premature database and must be regarded as preliminary in all relevant empirical respects. Moreover, in the absence of legislation on euthanasia, the general practice of dealing with patients on the edge of dying remains largely in a murky twilight zone. Since the late 1980s, there has been a public debate about euthanasia (*anlesi*, "peaceful death"), and many concerned doctors, ethicists, and social workers have raised the issue of treating dying patients humanely. However, this general awareness has not led to talking about death rationally.

This chapter intends to shed light on the current situation in China, with a special focus on the promising changes evolving in this field. If it should happen to provoke objections or criticism for being incomplete, or stimulate others to enlarge its scope and solidity, that will be a welcome contribution to progress in this vast research field in China. Such a process is meaningful on an international scale, too, to illuminate the related ethical debates as well as to guide international cooperation. The authors hope to make it clear that China, under adverse conditions of economic pressure and social transformation, offers a humane and reasonable vision of a dignified life with a good death that should guide decision makers. This vision is not only enshrined in the books of traditional Chinese ethics or in the minds of a few dedicated people, but has begun to take root in relevant institutions, education, fund-raising, and many practical activities.

Increasingly, then, issues involving decisions at the end of life are becoming matters of public policy. Advances in medicine have the capacity to extend a life that is often burdened with poor emotional and social quality. In light of the aging populations, scarce health care resources, and an expanding array of lifesaving technologies, end-of-life decisions are becoming more problematic. Demographically, the size of the aging population in China is expanding. Like the situation in many developed countries, the increasing incidence of chronic diseases will complicate end-of-life decision making in the coming decades, especially in urban areas. Also, owing to the success of the program to reduce the number of births, the Chinese population ratio is now out of balance. There are fewer productive people to provide the means to sustain a larger number of elderly. Moreover, in the cities, especially, there is evidence that the self-sustaining family-clan structures are collapsing. Family ties, once so stable, have begun to disintegrate. As a result, new concepts, such as solidarity, responsibility, and selfless care for others beyond the bounds of blood relatedness, will have to be introduced in order to maintain cohesive human structures in Chinese society.

This chapter examines how terminally ill and dying patients are and ought to be treated within the health care system in China. For reasons of data accessibility, the expertise of the contributors, and the special role the capital plays for China, Beijing was chosen as the focal region. However, in discussing what needs to be done in China (conceptually, ethically, and institutionally), end-of-life care is assessed from the perspective of a humanitarian framework. This reference scheme is influenced by the moral resources in present and traditional Chinese culture and tries to learn from the relevant international state of the art.

This chapter also introduces to an international readership concepts and guidelines that are proposed for the particular design of care for the terminally ill in China from the viewpoint of Chinese experts. It is written both as an account of the debate that is taking place in contemporary China on these issues and as a contribution to this same debate. Thus it attempts to be more than just a neutral piece of academic work, but argues for the merits of taking a position in fundamental matters of ethics in practice. The authors are aware that such a stand may easily expose the weaknesses of a humanitarian approach under conditions of economic and scientific globalization and the dominant spirit of competitiveness. This possibility notwithstanding, we hope that international and domestic readers will respond in sympathetic ways, offering constructive suggestions to improve the scholarship of research on end-of-life care issues in China on the moral grounds provided here.

The Concept of End-of-Life Care

The term "end-of-life care" (*linzhong guanhuai*) in China has the same original meaning as the English term "hospice care," which refers to those special places that accept incurable dying patients. We may also translate "hospice" into *anxisuo*, "place of peaceful rest." At its base, end-of-life care aims to help dying patients. The purpose is not to lengthen the patient's life span, but to improve the patient's quality of life. This includes looking after the patients, relieving their psychological problems, and comforting them. It makes greater efforts to control and ease their pain, soothing the anxiety and terror of death for patients and their family members. In this way, it is hoped, it maintains the dignity of patients and lets them die easily in comfort.

End-of-life care has emerged from a historical process. The ways we face death have developed over the course of millenia. Each individual's life is doomed to move toward death from the moment of birth. Our ancestors, when facing this reality, wanted to save life. They tried many methods to pursue an eternal life, which in the end proved to be impossible. Therefore, many kinds of myth were created to comfort humanity. Finally, it had to be admitted that death is unavoidable. In our times, humanity has begun to regard death in a more objective way, thus raising these concerns over care at the end of life.

More than 2000 years ago, China established "the asylum" (*bihu*) which is an embryonic form of the hospice. Later, the *yangbingfang*, *anjifang*, *pushan*, and *jiujiyuan* appeared, designed to look after patients and the elderly. These special organizations admitted elderly people who were disabled or had no kin and could not support themselves, as well as those who were too poor to sustain their daily lives. They offered little in the way of medical care, but when the old passed away, the organization would take charge of the funerals. These organizations were publicly supported through different government levels.

Since the early 1980s, measures have been taken to introduce formal end-of-life care and this has brought the matter to society's attention. From 1988 onward, Chinese academic circles have started to explore this field, and specialized hospitals such as the Beijing Songtang End of Life Care Hospice, Tianjin Medical University's End of Life Care Research Center, Shanghai City's Nanjiang Community Retired Employees Nursing Hospital, and Beijing Chaoyangmen Hospital's Second Ward (End of Life Care Ward) have been established. Moreover, the founding of community hospitals, community health services, and family hospital wards is also changing the tradition of "dying a natural death" in one's own home. In addition, the Beijing Academy for Medical Ethics has created an end-of-life committee, and research and scientific exchanges about end-of-life care have been initiated. Beijing, Tianjin, and other places have separately discussed these issues with experts in other countries. In a word, all of these steps have established a promising foundation for the growth of end-of-life care in China.

However, even though the debate over care at the end of life in its modern form was introduced in China more than 20 years ago, to the public and even many medical personnel, it is still a strange concept that they find difficult to understand. Some traditional views of life and death, as discussed later, have become cultural obstacles blocking scientific approaches to the dying process. Despite the improvements, there remain only a few hospitals specializing in end-of-life care, and they are in want of specialized technical personnel and proper medical standards. Furthermore, there are no adequate protocols for managing those clinics.

Today, among the top-ranking polyclinics of Beijing City there are only a few hospitals with dedicated end-of-life wards, and the community health services cannot satisfy the increasing demand. Also, as a result of the influence of a traditional death culture, such care is regarded as a family matter.

The new approach to end-of-life care is a great challenge for China. The aging population and the related change in causes of death indicate that it is important to increase efforts to enhance care at the end of life. In China the population that is 60 years and above is growing by 3.2 percent annually and by 2025 it will reach about 280 million or 18.4 percent of the total population. Furthermore, in 2050 it will reach about 400 million, that is, more than a quarter of the population. The arrival of the "old age society" increases the pressure on the rest of society to support the elderly and it makes end-of-life issues of vital importance.

It is a basic responsibility and also a historical mission for medical experts to create an end-of-life care system. The essential purpose of this system should be clear: Either the society or the household should take more responsibility for the old since their demands and dependence on society grow as they age. In view of this and drawing upon the experience of others in the field, we propose an approach that can be called a "One-Three-Nine pattern," which delineates one focal point, three perspectives, and nine connections.

One Focal Point
The main goal at the heart of all efforts is to relieve the patient's pain. Just before the end of life many patients suffer from extreme and unbearable pain. The use of analgesics, e.g., morphine, should take as a starting point the patient's needs and the state must back this up with the appropriate policy. In relieving the pain, we maintain the patient's dignity and allowing him or her to die in an easy and peaceful way, the best way to show our respect. Moreover, this approach to end-of-life care can help to reduce the family members' spiritual, psychological, and economic burden. It can also save labor and material resources for society by distributing resources more reasonably and promoting economic development. First, releasing family members from care may increase the productivity of society. Second, it undoubtedly saves health care

resources. Although to date there are no firm statistical data to support this assumption, the authors feel that such changes will eventually support healthy economic development.

Three Perspectives

End-of-life care hospitals, communal end-of-life services, and wards for family care at the end of life can be organized in a coordinated way and included in national public health and regional health plans. It is argued that all cities should establish end-of-life-care hospitals. For example, in large cities, six to eight hospitals with 80 to 120 beds each would be appropriate, and in medium-sized cities, establishing three to five hospitals is reasonable. A special end-of-life care hospital should have medical personnel, clinicians, psychologists, nurses, and a medical ethics committee composed of physicians and nursing experts, ethicists, a psychologist, a lawyer, and a manager.

With respect to the particular services to be offered in end-of-life units, the location, environment, and sanitation should be designed with special attention and the different units should support each other. As to the responsible health service administrative unit, the cities should establish basic health services for a specific block of streets, whereas the countryside depends on village and town hospitals. Today, regional health programming has re-formed the former mid- or mini-type hospitals into special geriatrics units. Given the current lack of specialized end-of-life hospitals, more attention should be given to the construction of family-supported wards for the terminally ill in these hospitals.

Nine Connections

The state, communities, and individuals must work together to provide service. Moreover, the service system must be built according to Chinese characteristics. This is a huge task for the entire society. The state should establish relevant policies, regulations, and laws and then put them into practice accordingly. It is also important to mobilize the local people. The Legal System's Collected Documents Journal (*Fazhi wenji bao*) has reprinted a report of the Anhui Daily (*Anhui Ribao*), that states:

According to related statistics, in China there are 2,816 institutions for social welfare organized by the government so far. They have 220,000 beds, of which 170,000 are occupied. In addition, 37,000 institutions organized by collectives have 870,000 beds, of which 660,000 are occupied in total. Compared to hundreds of millions of people who need social welfare in our country, the number of beds available now is just a little more than 0.7 percent. Less than 0.6 percent (of the population) has been admitted (to a hospital bed). That means we are far away from the developed countries, where 5 to 7 percent are admitted by welfare institutions. (*Anhui Ribao*, October 15, 2002)

Meeting the costs of end-of-life care will require financial support from the state, community, and society, as well as charity associations and donations by individual persons. The country should set up special funds to support end-of-life care work. At the same time, we should appeal to social groups and individuals to donate funds, establish special foundations, and guarantee the fund's regular use. Not the least, reforms of the medical insurance system need to be promoted.

In order to mobilize society to carry out the required measures and gradually build an adaptable framework, public awareness and knowledge about dying-related issues must be expanded. In the medical colleges and universities, classes on death and end-of-life care must be added, thus gradually creating a group of experts in these areas. Care for the terminally ill should be built up as an academic research subject to strengthen our understanding of, for example, traditional views of life and death, such as Confucian, Daoist, Buddhist, or Christian views. It should also include the philosophy of death, studies in human nature, medical concepts and purposes, euthanasia, patients' rights, social and economic aspects of death, and other topics. Academics have a responsibility to provide information for the end-of-life care regulations and to submit standards for protocols in dedicated units.

It is also important to establish a workable system for living wills and advance directives. On the basis of these measures, we can hope to make end-of-life decisions in practice more scientific and ethically sound on the levels of treatment, operations, and management.

Traditional Chinese Views of Death

Confucian Views

China is a country with a long history and a highly esteemed culture. Within this culture, Confucian ethics dominated China for more than 2000 years. Until the present, it has had a profound influence on the

Chinese people.[1] Even today Confucian views on death influence people's views to an extent that should not be underestimated.

Confucianism is traced back to Kong Zi (Confucius, 551–479 B.C.) in the later Spring and Autumn period (722–481 B.C.). It gradually took over the main stream of traditional culture in China, i.e., the feudalistic state doctrine that dominated academic thinking. Confucians generally believe that a life that has been fulfilled is the most precious thing for a human being and that not tolerating harm to one's parents is the fulfillment of filial piety.

Confucians believe that life and death have their allotted time; that all (true) wealth and honors are in heaven, and that human fate cannot be entrusted to spiritual entities. Confucius' and Meng Zi's "Doctrine of Heavenly Order" holds that a person's life and death are controlled by the resolve of one's expression of a natural moral sense. When people face their "Heavenly Order" they appear powerless.[2] This is the first characteristic of the Confucian view of death.

The second characteristic is that Confucians should not fear death if they have led a life of moral self-refinement. As Kong Zi states: "Everyone must die and the dead must be buried in the ground" (Chen Leping 1991: 74). "If I listen to the Dao in the morning, I will not be afraid of dying in the afternoon" (*Lunyu* 4.8). Meng Zi adds: "Through knowing our Heart we understand our Nature. By understanding our Nature we conceive Heaven. By preserving our Heart and nourishing our Nature, we can serve Heaven. By avoiding premature or artificially delayed death and pursuing the cultivation of ourselves, we may establish our lives upon the Heavenly Order" (*Mengzi*, 7A1). From this we can conclude that Confucians believe that in life human beings should submit to their duties and cultivate themselves according to good human nature so that they will not have to fear death and what lies beyond.

The third characteristic that Confucianism advocates is that we are to devote our lives to gaining humaneness (*ren*), as expressed in the phrase "to give up life in order to gain righteousness" (*she sheng qu yi*) (*Mengzi* 6 A 6). The *Lunyu* (in chapter 15.8) states: "The determined scholar and the man of virtue will not seek to live at the expense of injuring their virtue. They will even sacrifice their lives to preserve their virtue complete" (translation from Legge 1971: 297). Mengzi elsewhere states: "I desire to live, and I desire righteousness, too. In case that I cannot sustain both, I rather give up life and prefer righteousness" (*Mengzi* 6 A 10). The great compiler of the Confucian system of the Han dynasty, Dong Zhongshu (179–104 B.C.), also highlights: "For a gentleman, to live in disgrace is worse than to die in dignity" (Zhang 1988: 149).

In summary, Confucian views on death traditionally have played an important role in China. Respecting a person's life, not fearing death, and devoting life to gain honor are also important and valuable in modern Chinese society. However, the assumed Confucian attitude of meeting one's fate with submission is not appropriate today, but instead constitutes one of the major conceptual obstacles in dealing with euthanasia.

Daoist Views

Daoism (Taoism) has absorbed Confucian theories to form the main body of its religious moral view. Daoism is mainly represented by Lao Zi (Lao-tzu) and Zhuang Zi (350–280 B.C.). Lao Zi believes that "We enter (our lives) through being born, and we exit through death" (*Daodejing*, chapter 50; cf. Chan 1963 for a different translation). This describes the natural course of nature, which submits all humans, all creatures, and all affairs to the ceaseless transformation of the world. Everyone should accept this universal natural change. Death is a normal part of life, and we should accept it as a natural ordinance, a factual event we can do nothing about but accept.

It is impossible to avoid death and have an eternal life. In the *Daodejing*, Lao Zi states:

Three out of ten (people) are companions of life. Three out of ten are companions of death. And three out of ten in their lives lead from activity to death. And for what reason? Because of their vivid striving after life. I have heard that the one (of those ten) is a good preserver of his life and will not expose himself to tigers or wild buffaloes, and in fighting will not try to escape from weapons of war. And for what reason? Because in him there is no room for death. (*Daodejing*, chapter 50; quoted in Chan 1963: 163).

According to Daoist doctrine, in the special person's (accomplished man's) life, living and dying are shared equally. People may try their best to keep alive, but everyone is on the road to death. So we should view death as a kind of change that is part of nature's huge transformation.

The less we think about our own fear of death, the more we can touch the real nature of life. Thus we can surpass the limitation and anxiety of both death and life.

It is well known in China that when the wife of the second great Daoist philosopher, Zhuang Zi, died, instead of crying, he would chant a song and beat his drum. His friend and philosophical opponent, Hui Zi, accused him, saying "You couple have lived together for a long time. Now your wife has passed away, but you never show any grief, but sing a song and beat the drum!" Zhuang Zi replied,

This is not true. At first moment, I was so sad, but then I thought about it. Once she had had no life, no form, and no energy; but then, in the limbo of existence and non-existence, owing to the transformation, her energy was created, followed by her form and then by her coming to life. Now she has been transformed again, from the living to the dead. It is like the season's turning. So now my wife rests in the great hall of Heaven and Earth. Why should I cry any more? If I had continued moaning, I really would not have understood the principle of life and death. So I will never feel sad. [*Zhuangzi*, "Zhi Le" ("On Greatest Happiness"), abridged; translation and comment in Chan 1963: 209).

Buddhist Views

Buddhism started to appear in the fifth and sixth centuries B.C. and spread from India to China. The Indian concept of a Buddha is a person who understands the truth. Early Buddhism's basic religious doctrine is called "Explanation of the Four Divine Offerings" (*Si di shuo*). This refers to kudi, jidi, miedi and the daodi as the "four offerings." In this doctrine, "*kudi*" means that we should look on the real world with a sublime eye. The real world is not perfect, but full of afflictions and illusions, which concretely include the pain of living, aging, sickening, and dying, and even the concept of personal individuality (*anâtman*) (Keown 1995). "*Jidi*" indicates that the cause of all sufferings is our urgent aspiration for happiness, because it binds us to illusion and should be overcome. "*Miedi*" is a higher state of insight in which these aspirations are all dissolved together with the associated consciousness. The fourth "offering," "*daodi*," is to approach the highest stage in a Buddhist's life, by preparing to enter Nirvana.

Buddhism espouses *Samsara* and transmigration of souls. According to these ideas, doing the good thing will establish a good *Kharma* (acquired fate), which is expected to contribute to a good life in the next incarnation. On the other hand, a sinful life causes a bad start for the next incarnation, and makes overcoming the circle of living and dying less likely. Buddhists believe that in the present era, no one can have a happy life, because true happiness is beyond the realm of illusion. Hence, they do not fear dying as much as the odds of being reborn.

Many people fear death and are afraid that their individual existence could vanish. Some fear that their death will have a distressing influence on their family members. Quite a few fears are related to superstitious beliefs. Some people fear death because they might never finish their business in life. However, others do not fear death because they know it cannot be avoided. More important, for many Buddhists in particular, death without suffering means the chance to enter a new life, or even to escape the wheel of incarnations. Some people think death is an opportunity, and that it is the proper time to leave the "circle of life." Others think that the meaning of death can be explained in terms of meaningfulness and purpose. Some people, especially Buddhists and Daoists, are unafraid of death because they expect their spiritual self to be eternal.

Moral Principles in End-of-Life Care

While those who need care at the end of life form a special group of people, they should still be considered as patients. They may appear to be hopelessly drifting in an endless sea, fearing to drown at any time, but because these patients are on the verge of death, they need more love and care at this time. This is why medical personnel should observe not only general medical ethics principles but also ethical principles that are particularly relevant at the end of life.

Medical Humanism

Humanism (*rendao zhuyi*) is a world view that cares for the human being, respects it, and places it in the center of attention. In China, during the Spring and Autumn period (722–481 B.C.), the Warring States period (403–222 B.C.), and influenced by ancient philosophical thinking and ethics, medical humanism developed. The Confucian "humane affection" (*ren ai*), the Mohist's[3] "universal love and mutual benefit," (*jian ai hu li*), and the Daoist "the lasting virtue is not remote" (*chang de bu li*) are examples. The *Huangdi Neijing* says "Among all covered by Heaven and carried by Earth, among the entirety of all things and beings: nothing is as valuable as the human" (quoted in Unschuld 2003: 19).

During the twentieth century, medical humanism was developed further. Many statements, declarations, and guidelines acknowledge that sustaining people's health is most important. In 1975, the twenty-ninth meeting of the World Medical Association passed "the Tokyo Declaration," which stated that "in any situation, a doctor may not support, tolerate, or participate in maltreatment or inhumane behavior." Medical humanism advocates caring for and sympathizing with the patient. An example of this principle is Beijing Songtang Hospital, where the staff treats the dying patients around the clock as if they were their own family. In addition, volunteers from the Capital University of Medical Sciences set up a "love cabin" (*aixin xiaowu*) where they visit patients regularly, chat with them, sing for them, comb their hair, and trim their fingernails.

Informed Consent

All citizens in China have the right to self-determination, within the boundaries of the law. A patient in care at the end of life has the legal right to accept or reject a proposed treatment. If the patient is mentally competent, the medical personnel should respect the patient's decision. If the patient is unable to make a decision because of incapacity, the medical personnel may act according to the patient's advance directive (*yuzhu zhixing*), should one exist. Since September 2002, a set of "Regulations of Conflicts in Medical Treatment" (*Yiliao shigu chuli tiaoli*) has been in effect in China. The first clause defines the purpose of the regulations: "[T]o sort out claims after medical accidents, to protect the legal rights of both the patients and the medical institution and its personnel, to safeguard the medical system, to ensure medical safety and to promote the development of the medical sciences." Clause 10 points out that patients have the right to obtain and copy their medical records, the doctor's advice record, laboratory test and imaging test records, any agreements to undergo diagnostic tests or surgery, the record of the procedure as well as the anesthesia, records of pathological tests, nursing records, and others as specified by the government. These regulations are prescribed as national statutes to protect the rights of all patients.

Respect for the End of Life

Respect is a fundamental moral principle. It is the unconditional moral duty of medical personnel to respect all patients, including those at the end of life. Only when medical personnel respect the patients and their family members can mutual trust be created. Medical personnel should respect the needs of the dying patients as expressed by their choice of medical treatment, their faith, and their preferred manner of death.

Compassion

The principle of compassion (*guanhuai*) is critical at the end of life because patients can be undergoing extreme suffering. Compassion includes relieving pain, providing appropriate care, and helping the dying patient deal with psychological problems. Medical personnel should also have compassion for the family members of a dying patient and provide emotional support. Given enough time, doctors can instruct family members on how to care for the patient, thus helping family members prepare for their loved one's death and fulfill their moral duties, thereby giving them relief from sorrow when the patient passes away.

Development of End-of-Life Care in Hospitals

Starting service in 1990, the Beijing Songtang Hospital is a well-known hospital for end-of-life care. The hospital pledges to try its best to let patients pass away without sorrow. From its founding, Songtang was the first to actualize a comprehensive medical concept based on a belief that patients are the center of medical treatment. Songtang offers psychological care; 93 percent of its patients have no religious belief and most of them refuse to face the fact that they are dying. Being familiar with this mindset, the doctors treat them individually and warmly, paying much attention to their psychic and religious needs. Songtang Hospital has received delegates from 236 medical organizations, social institutions, and individuals from all over the country, including provinces of Inner Mongolia, Xinjiang, and Hainan. Also, scholars and experts from thirty countries visited Songtang during its first 11 years, mainly to learn about the psychological care its staff offers to dying patients.

Beijing Chaoyangmen Hospital's End of Life Care ward was founded in July 1992. Independent from the hospital, this ward specializes in social medicine in Beijing City. The ward admits patients who are sick from various causes, including natural infirmity, organ failure, frailty, cerebrovascular disease, accidental injury, cancer, and terminal stages of chronic illnesses. The dedication of the personnel in serving the spiritual wellsprings of life marks this ward as a pioneer in this field. As an institution that combines medicine, nursing, scientific research, teaching, and voluntary service, it was constructed primarily as a window to the world of the city's community service.

Hong Kong's Baipuli Ningji Center, established in 1986, is located in Shatin in the New Territories. Its main purpose is to provide end-of-life care to residents from Hong Kong and the adjacent regions. Care is offered to both the dying patient and his or her family. The center was initially financed through private projects and corporations and is dedicated to providing comprehensive care at the end of life. Terminal cancer patients can enjoy self-respect, feel at home, and come to the close of their lives serenely. The motto of the center is "Our life-span is endowed by Heaven, while our life's meaning is achieved by the human being."

In addition to these centers, other institutions and individual endeavors in end-of-life care are emerging, and they are accompanied by increasing efforts in related research. For example, Tianjin Medical University set up an End of Life Care Center in July 1988, and established wards in October 1990. In the same year, a new hospital dedicated to such care, Nanhui Huliyuan, came into existence in Shanghai, and the Academy of Medical Ethics in Beijing created a special committee for end-of-life care. During the following years, similar facilities appeared in Xi'an and in Shenyang. In China, there are currently approximately 100 service organizations for end-of-life care. In parallel, theoretical research is improving through experience in practice. Having obtained support from both the government and the citizens, the progress is promising.

Trends of End-of-Life Care in China

The hospice theory in China was developed on the basis of Confucianism, Buddhism, Daoism, and traditional ethics, with typical East Asian cultural features. Human beings are influenced in the development of their thinking by the environment in which they live. When people have to live in an unhealthy environment, the requirements of survival come first. Only when people live under conditions of peace and abundance can they develop higher cultural aspirations (Arendt 1958). It is difficult for human beings to strive for refined culture when their lives are in constant danger and they lack basic necessities.

The improved economic environment in most modern societies means that these societies can now provide higher levels of care for dying patients; more of their needs can be satisfied and their quality of life improved. One purpose of studying end-of-life care is to determine the patients' true needs, and how patients are affected by their varied backgrounds, such as living experiences, cultural upbringing, and religious beliefs. Another purpose is to enable hospice staff to provide more scientific and attentive care for the dying patient.

From the beginning, the end-of-life debate in China has sparked imaginative approaches that can enrich the global hospice movement. While learning from Western hospice theories, researchers and staff are working hard in researching and developing a Chinese hospice theory using an approach that combines theory and practice. Some end-of-life care hospitals and medical agencies are trying to improve their skills by enlarging the range of their practice, reinforcing discussion of theory, and strengthening exchange and cooperation programs with other countries. At present, China is communicating with the United States, Germany, Japan, Hong Kong, and Taiwan about end-of-life policies. Beijing City already offers special hospitals for the elderly in every district, and it is envisaged that there will be at least one institution in every district and county in China by 2005.

Relieving Pain

Medical scholars have suggested that the average period of dying for a terminal patient is 6 months. However, the results of clinical observation of nearly 8,000 patients conducted by Beijing Songtang Hospital indicate that the time from irreversible deterioration of health to death for about 90 percent of the patients is actually about 10 months. While the dying process has both physiological and psychic stages, for the majority of patients, the physiological and psychic degenerations do not take place synchronously. Physiological dying is characterized by the degeneration of organs and systems, which leads to an inability to care for oneself and makes it necessary to seek help from the nursing staff, with the application of various measures, medical equipment, or medicines. For about 75 percent of patients, the physiological dying period is over before the psychological dying period begins. This extends from the onset of unclear consciousness to the end of life.

Many dying patients, especially cancer patients, are in severe pain, which puts an enormous stress on the patient's body and soul, affecting both quality of life and dignity. Simultaneously, the patient's family members are also heavily affected. In trying to relieve pain and provide comfort, it is important to note that the degree of pain may vary from person to person and according to their ethnic identity. Research and production of medicines and medical procedures for pain relief should be designed in a way that considers individual and ethnic differences. Also, special spiritual exercises can be helpful in relieving pain.

Psychological Treatment at the End of Life
For a nursing staff, the first thoughts when facing a patient are "How can I understand her or him? How can I relieve this patient's fear and anxiety? I must try to shorten the distance between us; she or he is a friend who needs our help." Flexible and effective psychological measures must be taken to relieve pain and reduce psychological stress according to the needs of different individuals, who may react to their illness with fear, evasion, resisting treatment, or passively waiting for death. Research that improves our understanding of the process of dying is important to make psychological treatment at the end of life more effective. The extent to which patients' requirements are fulfilled is a criterion in the evaluation of hospices. Demands should be satisfied as much as possible, while considering that needs may vary among persons. However, even when natural and social environments and cultures differ,

the guarantee of human rights, the desire to be loved, and the need to be cared for are universal.

In summary, the purpose and science of end-of-life care have a unique appeal. A hospice makes it possible for staff members and social workers to engage in a fulfilled life with the dying patients under their care while supporting each patient's dignity. However, there still is a gap between what has been accomplished and the ultimate goals. For example, in clinical practice, it is difficult to comprehend what the patient really needs. Also, since medical staff members often are not familiar with psychological care, more attention and efforts are needed to improve psychological care.

Euthanasia

People are like reeds, the most awe-inspiring life in nature; at the same time, they are like pensive reeds. If you want to destroy someone, you won't need to use the power of the whole universe, but a puff of smoke or a drop of water is enough.
—Li Yiting

On January 3, 1994, Chen Li, a young peasant in a small county in Jiangsu Province, strangled her husband, Du Haizhi, who was terminally ill with liver cancer. Because the couple loved each other dearly, Chen Li couldn't bear to watch her beloved suffer from the severe pain. Du Haizhi, who could not tolerate the pain any longer, had asked the doctor in charge of his case to help him to pass away, but he refused. Then Chen Li, motivated by love and compassion for her husband, took action. After Du died, his brother's wife filed a lawsuit against Chen. She was declared guilty and spent 3 years in prison based on Section 132 in Chinese criminal law. This case provoked enraged comments from all over the country and invited reconsideration of whether euthanasia should be made legal in China (Yu and Shi 1998).

The Concept of Euthanasia
The English term "euthanasia" goes back to the Greek expression for "good death," and originally meant "dying without pain." From the viewpoint of medical methods, we can distinguish between passive and

active euthanasia. In passive euthanasia, hopeless treatment is discontinued at the request of the patient or his or her family, allowing the patient to die naturally in order to stop the pain; hence it is called "to let die" (*tingren siwang*). Some clinics in China have implemented this method. In active euthanasia, steps are taken to hasten the dying process. It is called "mercy assisted dying" (*renci zhusi*).

Active euthanasia is sometimes translated as "the art of causing death without pain." As such, it is seen as the process of comforting patients with incurable diseases so that their dying stage is without pain. The patient's accelerated death should not be the direct result of this treatment, but might be acceptable on balance as a side effect of reducing the suffering (double effect). It must be pointed out that *anlesi* is driven by a the desire to comfort the patient during the dying process.

From the viewpoint of a patient, euthanasia can be classified as voluntary (*ziyuan*) or involuntary (*fei ziyuan*) cases (Lo 1999, 2001). In voluntary euthanasia, the patient requests euthanasia, either directly if capable or indirectly by asking others to do so according to an advance directive. Involuntary euthanasia involves patients who have no such ability, such as infants and comatose or mentally ill persons. These patients are not able to explain their wishes adequately and have no advance directive, and the question of whether to execute euthanasia can be decided only by the doctors. Although it is described academically, it is illegal to commit involuntary euthanasia in China and it is thus strictly forbidden in clinical practice.

The essence of *anlesi* is not to make a decision about life and death, but rather to determine whether someone must die in agony or in peace. Its objective is to ameliorate the dying process by reducing the pain of spirit and body through the consolation and help offered by medical management and control.

In China, the first euthanasia symposium was held in Shanghai in 1988 (Qiu 1999). In December 1994, an article, "Death of a Doctor," was published in the Chinese journal *Health News* (*Jiankangbao*) and recommended euthanasia in the case of Zhao Xunmei, a cancer patient at Shanghai Huadong Hospital who ultimately killed herself. Obviously, there exists a quiet practice of euthanasia in China. Surveys conducted by Guo Qingxiu and Ying Yi and Li Yiting in 1987 and 1988 found that, respectively, 62.6 and 79.8 percent of the public supported euthanasia. At present, pain alleviation is the main treatment available for dying patients in China. There are no clear standards or indicators for withdrawing active therapy because, to date China has not formally made the related laws. The Chinese government has had discussions about a euthanasia law, but no conclusion has been reached (Du 2002).

The Ethical Debate over Euthanasia

In 1986, a 59-year-old female patient named Xia was hospitalized in Hanzhong City, Shanxi Province, with symptoms of cirrhosis of the liver and edema of the abdomen. During treatment, the patient was frightened and hysterical. She was only able to calm down and sleep after being injected with a tranquilizer. When her son and daughter learned from the doctor that their mother could not be cured because of the late stage of her liver disease, they several times expressed their wish to stop their mother's life "to save her from pain and suffering." They said that they were willing to take all the responsibility. This situation gave rise to legal disputes after the patient had passed away. There are many cases of patient suicide and some cases of doctors actively killing, or assisting patients to commit suicide (Zhai 1998). In his book, *Suicide and Life*, He Zhaoxiong estimates that 20 to 40 percent of the patients in hospital have suicidal thoughts and 2 percent have a suicidal determination (1996).

Debates about the advantages and disadvantages of euthanasia have continued without reaching a conclusion (Shen, 2002). Generally, four arguments against euthanasia are cited. First, all life is sacred; the right to live is a person's most fundamental right. The duty of doctors is only to save patients, and to prolong their lives. Second, a doctor's diagnosis and prognosis cannot always be 100 percent correct, and advanced science and technology may bring hope to patients with formerly "incurable diseases." Third, it is difficult to determine whether a patient's decision to die is voluntary. Fourth, euthanasia can amount to "treating human life as grass" (*caojian renming*; i.e., not to account for the value of human life), making it in consequence like murder.

In contrast, five arguments are commonly cited in support of euthanasia. First, the sanctity of life is not limited to a right to live, but also includes a right to die. Second, it is more important to relieve the pain than to prolong the life of a dying patient in unbearable pain. Third, in many cases a patient's will can be determined, for example by an advance directive. Fourth, aside from considering a patient's benefit, we should also consider the public's interest, including community welfare and the value of resources; it is wasteful to spend considerable resources to save a life without meaning. Fifth, the arrival of new technology should not be used as an excuse for ignoring dying people's suffering; moreover, we are not sure whether such technology will actually appear.

In theoretical discussions and ethical and moral analysis, the implementation of some kind of *anlesi*/euthanasia can certainly be justified. However, in clinical practice, when performing acts of euthanasia, physicians should insist on a conceptual framework of the sanctity and quality of life and cherish harmony of life values. We must insist on the ethical principles of beneficence, voluntarity, and justice. In this view, standards must be strictly controlled so that all practical procedures are covered by the regulations. Appropriate laws and regulations are needed, and specialized committees must monitor the practice of euthanasia.

Views of the End of Life

The body of him who has walked a long road is weak. He lacks the strength to walk even one more step. He has taken the entire heavy burden from his shoulders; he feels relaxed as he had never felt before.
—Li Yiting

This is a story told by a doctor who witnessed a child's last days. "Jiemi was only eight. He was so unfortunate [as] to be infected by his father. During the three days before his death he went through two bad crises. I had to re-induce his heartbeat by electric stimulation. I still remember the moment when he encountered such a crisis again. I was preparing for the electric stimulator when Jiemi suddenly opened his eyes and asked me not to 'shun away' God. He told me that he was missing God indeed and life there was better than here, without pains and worries. Several days later, Jiemi went to that better world quietly" (Feng Chen, personal communication, 1991).

At all times and in all places, seeking a long life is a human trait. However, people usually avoid talking about death. In contrast to Jiemi, most people are terrified about death, and wish it would not happen, or at least that it could be delayed for as long as possible. A strong emotional reaction often occurs when old people learn that they are going to die. At first they will deny the prognosis vehemently; they simply won't have it that they must die. They cry all day and lament their bad fate. Only after telling their relatives and discussing the afterlife do they calm down again.

Fear and passivity have the power to destroy a tranquil life. Heavy psychological burdens hasten an early death. It is very important for old people to establish a proper attitude toward life and to restrain the fear of death and depression, since these latter two tendencies are harmful. We should let old people understand that science and reason offer ways to strengthen the body, resist decline, and prolong life, thus, possibly delaying the coming of death. Fear and passivity are not helpful. Life remains meaningful only if even a short existence is used for work, study, and cultural activities. We should be happy about life, and calm about death, "not let the heart die before the body dies."

Where Do People Die and Who Decides?

Owing to the influences of health policy and family morals, Chinese people choose different dying places, depending on their circumstances. In rural areas, many old people insist on dying at home, reflecting the belief that "falling leaves go back down to the roots." Even those who have received long-term therapy in a hospital will insist on coming home before death. Generally, residents in cities die in hospitals while those in the countryside die in a hospital or at home.

A lot of money is spent on dying patients in ordinary hospitals because of the higher demand for emergency treatment there. The expense for staying in a hospice is lower than in ordinary hospitals because treatment there is limited mostly to palliative care. According to statistical data from some hospital wards in Beijing, about 2,000 RMB (approximately $250US) are needed for a dying patient per month. This is more than many peasant families earn annually. This is about three times as much as the expenses in hospices. The expense for terminal patients in hospitals increases markedly during the last 3 to 6 months of life. However, in hospices there is no such obvious increase.

At present, among the many parties, including government, hospitals, and ethics committees, the family remains the most important factor in decision making at the end of life. Within the family, the father or head of a household has to make the decisions (*juece*) and has to take primary responsibility. In Chinese culture, it is customary for the family to make important decisions, with parents, generally speaking, playing the leading role in this process. Eventually, children will have a greater role because the decision-making procedure has become more democratic, and in some families, children already take a leading role. No matter which part of the household dominates, the whole family will carry out the decision.

The Experience of Facing Death and the Dying Process
Research on patients who had been diagnosed as terminally ill and recovered might help us understand the psychological reactions of an individual in an extreme crisis and the psychological changes that occur during the dying process. Some clinical reports have found that some patients changed positively after the experience of facing death. Afterward, they reported that they cherished life significantly more than earlier and displayed abundant energy and fresh vigor. E. Mansell Pattison, a psychiatrist who has studied the process of terminal illness, points out that in dying, people suffer from various kinds of dreadful experiences, such as loneliness, loss of self-control, out-of-body experiences, reversion, and so on (Nan Chuan 2001, referring to Pattison's views).

Not all patients experience extreme pain and anguish, or extreme fear. Also, not every patient shows serious bodily symptoms or a disturbed consciousness. At least some patients are clearly conscious before dying and understand what is happening. Usually they are calm, although they might have feelings of withdrawal, alienation, and isolation. Some patients are worried, hostile, angry, sad, struggling, and uncooperative.

Some researchers have found that close to the end of the dying period, the ability to hear deteriorates. However, family members are advised not to make noises, whisper to each other, or cry loudly so as not to disturb the process of the fading of the senses or inhibit "departure of the soul." An American scholar, Elisabeth Kubler-Ross, divided the psychological course between the moment a patient learns about his or her illness to the moment of death into five segments: denial and isolation, anger, bargaining, depression, and acceptance of death (Kubler-Ross 1969). Nan Chuan (a Chinese counterpart of Kubler-Ross) (2001), in the famous "experience death with celebrities" also points out that the spiritual awareness of death increases as the illness proceeds.

The condition for allowing a patient to accept the inevitability of death allows him to prepare for his departure, finalizing affairs and leaving them in good order for the family. This implies especially the right to be informed about the coming of death. Hence, it is the responsibility of doctors to explain the true nature of the dying process and try their best to help the dying person to cope with the situation. Many investigations show that the majority of patients expect to be informed accurately about the state of their illness, and to learn about the coming of death directly from their doctors. Of course, it is necessary for doctors to be sympathetic and have good interpersonal skills in informing the critically ill patient.

Real-life evidence shows that the most urgent need of most dying patients is to see their family members. In fact, in China's traditional cultural conception, "to attend upon the dying parents' bedside" occupied a very important position. A person who did not attend upon his dying parent would be labeled unfilial (Wang 1999). Furthermore, his personality, moral character, and level of cultivation might be suspected. Thus, the Chinese traditionally take attending the dying parents' bedside very seriously. As society changes and the market economy continues to develop, however, this concept is being affected. For example, aged parents often pass away unaccompanied, feeling sad about the impossibility of meeting their family members, because their children either live far away or are busy working. The nursing staff should inform the dying person's family members so that they may arrive at the bedside in time. In urgent situations, the doctor should do his best to prolong the dying of the patient if appropriate. Though the patient would have to endure pain, this prolonged suffering might be acceptable compared with the possible suffering from not meeting with his or her family members.

The Importance of Funerals in China

Mourning, burying the dead, and participating in memorial services provide important assistance in dealing with the death of others as well as our own. Tradition and customs can contribute to this process. Although funerals focus on the burial of the dead, for the survivors in Chinese culture, it is the aim to see that the dead are still present in loving and respectful ways. Chinese funerals tend to be clan funerals and people obey the burial regulations of their clan. According to the "The Great (Minister of Education) Si Tu on Matters of the Clan" from the "Classical Documents from the Zhou Dynasty" (*Zhouli*), burial regulation is one of six important customs. It states: "Arrange the tombs near to each other, so that people have the company of their relatives" (*fen mu xiang lian, min nai you qin*).

China's culture has guided and helped the Chinese since ancient times to cope with the crisis of death. Individuals are required to fully respect their parents all their lives. Every individual is inculcated with the moral relationships of loyalty and filial respect from the time of birth. From birth to death, there is not even a slight relaxation or release that would exempt someone from these duties.

Conclusion: Attention to End-of-Life Care

Decision making at the end of life will become much more humane, practical, rational and in accord with China's cultures if it is based on the concept of hospice care as described here. Before procedural regulations for implementing end-of-life decisions are drawn up, however, it is necessary to provide an adequate infrastructure, to introduce the related humanitarian concepts to the public, and to install a system of general education and special training to ensure the quality and sustainability of this project.

The provision of suitable care at the end of life contributes to the common good. It plays a significant role as part of health care reform in restructuring and developing Chinese society. The Chinese government must support and facilitate this project on all levels. Social organizations and individuals should join in making greater efforts to inform the public about the issues surrounding the end of life and the advantages of hospice care. Moreover, greater economic investment must be made to support existing institutions as well as to fund new initiatives. The aging of the population poses economic as well as social and individual challenges. As this population grows and the younger population declines in numbers, end-of-life care will play an increasingly important role in care of the elderly. To care for, respect, and love others is natural for a human being. Thus it is our responsibility to take part in care at the end of life, to promote this care, to improve people's health, and to transform society. The transformation of Chinese society takes place at all levels at the same time: economic, political, social, intellectual and cultural. Advancement is needed at all of these levels in order to provide the material and intellectual base for needed change. By building successful hospices as a small but important contribution to this process we can set examples for others, inside China and beyond.

Acknowledgments

The authors would like to thank the following persons for their contributions to this chapter: Li Fang, Wang Xueke, Fang Fang, and Chen Zhang.

Notes

1. The designations Confucianism, Daoism, and Buddhism in the following passages refer to the popular understandings of these moral traditions in the sense of Berger and Hsiao (1988) and MacFarquhar (1980), although they do not claim accuracy in scholarly terms. For the philosophical concepts and key texts, see Roetz (1993) and Chan (1963). For a contemporary Confucian approach to end-of-life care, see Döring (2001).

2. "When one does not know the Heavenly Order (*tian ming*), one can not become a Gentleman (*junzi*)" (*Lunyu* 20.3). Mencius (Meng Zi, 372–281 B.C.) says: "There is nothing without its proper order. We must humbly accept what has been ordered" (*Mengzi* 7 A 2). Meng Zi, otherwise known as Mencius, is the second great Confucian after Master Kong Fuzi (Confucius).

3. The philosophical school of Mo Di or Mo Zi (479–438 B.C.) was a major opponent to the Confucian schools, taking a utilitarian view.

References

Arendt, Hannah. 1958. *The Human Condition*. Chicago: University of Chicago Press.

Berger, Peter L., and Hsiao Hsin-Huang Michael, eds. 1988. *In Search of an East Asian Development Model.* New Brunswick, N.J.: Transaction.

Chan, Wing-tsit. 1963. *A Sourcebook in Chinese Philosophy.* Princeton, N.J.: Princeton University Press.

Chen, Leping. 1991. *Zhongguo Yixue Wenhua Daolun—Churu Mingmen.* Shanghai: Sanlian.

Döring, Ole. 2001. "The meaning of death and dying. Confucian reflections on quality of life assessment at the end of life." *Formosa Medical Ethics Journal* 2 (October): 48–66.

Du, Zhizheng. 2002. "An ethical defense of withdrawing medical treatment." In *Advances in Chinese Medical Ethics: Chinese and International Perspectives,* edited by Ole Döring and Renbiao Chen. Hamburg: Mitteilungen des Instituts für Asienkunde No. 355, pp. 306–314.

He, Zaoxiong. 1996. *Zisha yu Rensheng* (Suicide and Life). Guangzhou: Guangzhou Publishing House.

Keown, Damien. 1995. *Buddhism and Bioethics.* New York: St. Martins Press.

Kubler-Ross, Elisabeth. 1969. *On Death and Dying.* London: Macmillan.

Legge, James. 1971. *Confucius. Confucian Analects, The Great Learning and the Doctrine of the Mean.* New York: Dover.

Li, Yiting, and Wei Li. 2000. *Linzhongbing Huaixue* (Psychological Issues at the End of Life). Beijing: Zhongguo kexue zhisu chubanshe.

Lo, Ping-cheung. 1999. "Confucian views on suicide and their implications for euthanasia." In Fan Ruiping, *Confucian Bioethics,* Dordrecht, Netherlands: Kluwer, pp. 69–101.

Lo, Ping-cheung. 2001. "Zai Taishan yu emao zhi jian, rujia cunsheng qusi de jiashiguan" (Between Mount Tai and a swan's feather. A Confucian discussion of living and dying). *Zhongwai yixue zhexue* 3 (2): 5–50.

MacFarquhar, Roderick. 1980. "The post-Confucian challenge." *Economist* (February 9): 67–72.

Nan, Chuan (edited by Huang Tanping). 2001. *Yu Mingjia Yiqi Tiyan Si* (Understanding Death in the Spirit of Fate). Beijing: Guangming Daily Publishing House.

Qiu, Renzong. 1999. "Medical ethics in China: Status quo and main issues." In *Chinese Scientists and Responsibility,* edited by Ole Döring. Hamburg: Mitteilungen des Instituts für Asienkunde No. 314, pp. 24–32.

Roetz, Heiner. 1993. *Confucian Ethics of the Axial Age: A Reconstruction under the Aspect of the Breakthrough toward Postconventional Thinking.* Albany: State University of New York Press.

Shen, Mingxian. 2002. "Euthanasia and Chinese traditional culture." In *Advances in Chinese Medical Ethics: Chinese and International Perspectives,* edited by Ole Döring and Renbiao Chen. Hamburg: Mitteilungen des Instituts für Asienkunde No. 355, pp. 255–264.

Unschuld, Paul U. 2003. *The Huang Di Nei Jing Su Wen* (Nature, Knowledge, Imagery in an Ancient Chinese Medical Text). Berkeley: University of California Press.

Wang, Qingjie. 1999. "The Confucian filial obligation and care for aged parents." In *Confucian Bioethics*, edited by Fan Ruiping. Dordrecht, Netherlands: Kluwer, pp. 235–256.

Yu, Lin, and Shi Dajie. 1998. "It is necessary to legalize euthanasia in China: From public opinion polls and representative cases." *Zhongwai Yixue Zhexue* 1 (1): 16–29.

Zhai, Xiaomei. 1998. "Anlesi: Lunli he Gainian Wenti" (Euthanasia: Conceptual and Ethical Issues), Ph.D. thesis. Beijing: Chinese Academy of Social Sciences.

Zhang, Liping. 1988. *Zhongguo Wenhua gaixian* (Subtleties of Chinese Culture). Shanghai: Dongfang.

4

End-of-Life Decision Making in Germany

Alfred Simon

Developments in the Netherlands, especially the current law that regulates killing on demand and physician-assisted suicide, have once more started the debate on medical end-of-life decision making in Germany. Survey results show that the majority of the German population is in favor of a regulation similar to the one in the Netherlands. However, corresponding initiatives to extend existing laws in this direction have not been politically successful so far.

In the mid-1980s a group of professors of criminal law and medicine submitted an alternative draft bill on medical decisions at the end of life (Baumann et al. 1986). This draft did not intend to legalize killing on demand (in Germany called active euthanasia), but the courts were given the opportunity to forgo punishment under certain conditions. Furthermore, the draft contained paragraphs that were to specify when terminating or omitting a life-sustaining measure (so-called "passive euthanasia"), administering pain-relieving drugs with the result of hastening death (so-called "indirect euthanasia"), and not preventing suicide would not be unlawful—three areas that are not explicitly regulated by German law so far (see the section on legal regulations and court decisions).

In May 1985, a public hearing on the topic took place before the Legal Affairs Committee of the German Bundestag. The majority of the invited experts were of the opinion that active euthanasia should be rejected on principle and that there was no need for further legal regulation. The majority of the attendees at the 56th German Jurists Forum also voted against the legal regulation of medical decisions at the end of life.

Current controversies and conflicting court decisions—e.g., on the termination of artificial feeding and fluid supply in coma patients—show, however, that contrary to the opinion of many experts at that time, the problems in question can no longer be solved adequately simply by an interpretation of the law that is in force. This especially concerns the boundaries between active and passive euthanasia.

The need for legal regulation of the different forms of euthanasia and the current debate about it are described in the second part of this chapter. The first part presents basic facts and numbers on death and dying in Germany. Finally a summary is given and conclusions are drawn.

The Situation of Dying People in Germany

In Germany, debates about medical end-of-life decision making are mostly held on a theoretical basis. Empirical data—especially on deaths outside the hospital—are frequently not known or nonexistent. It is indicative of the situation that Germany is not represented in the two current projects on end-of-life decision making supported by the European Union (ETHICATT and End-of-Life Decision, see http://www.cordis.lu). In this chapter the situation of dying people in Germany is described using the available data. First, relevant epidemiological and economic data are presented, and then the existing supply structures for palliative care are examined.

Epidemiological Data

In Germany, 838,797 persons died in the year 2000. Nearly half of the deaths were caused by diseases of the cardiovascular system, particularly in older people (approximately 90 percent of the deceased were more than 65 years old). About a quarter of all the deceased died from cancer. Of the 11,100 persons who committed suicide in the year 2000, 74 percent were men and 26 percent women. Nearly half of all deaths took place in hospitals; there was hardly any change in the percentage of those who died in hospitals from 1991 to 2000 (table 4.1).

No reliable details can be given about the places of death outside the hospital. While the place of death is stated on the official death certificate, data are neither collected centrally nor analyzed statistically. Moreover, legal regulations concerning data protection restrict a review of

Table 4.1
Deaths in Germany, 1991 to 2000

Year	Total numbers of deaths	Deaths in hospitals	
		Number	Percent of total
1991	911,245	444,936	48.8
1992	885,443	436,954	49.3
1993	897,270	440,176	49.1
1994	884,661	429,005	48.5
1995	884,588	424,910	48.0
1996	882,843	414,129	46.9
1997	860,389	403,560	46.9
1998	852,382	402,962	47.3
1999	846,330	403,462	47.7
2000	838,797	402,912	48.0

Source: Federal Statistical Office Germany, http://www.destatis.de.

death certificates. This explains why only a few regionally and temporally limited surveys on places of death outside hospitals exist in Germany (Hoffmann and Adolph 2001).

The most extensive survey on this topic so far dates from the year 1997 and concerns persons who died in the German state of Rhineland-Palatinate in 1995 (Ochsmann et al. 1997). Since the results of this survey correspond to a large degree with the results of subsequent surveys carried out in other German states (cf. Bickel 1998; van Oorschot et al. 2002), it may be assumed that the data for Rhineland-Palatinate are fairly representative of the current situation in Germany (table 4.2).

With 44 percent of all deaths, the hospital was the most significant place of dying in Rhineland-Palatinate in the year 1995. Also, nearly 13 percent of all deaths took place in nursing homes. All in all, about 57 percent of the persons recorded died in institutions. However, approximately 40 percent of all persons died in private homes, which is significantly more than is generally assumed. With increasing age, the percentage of persons who died in nursing homes rose from about 3 percent in the 60–69-year-old group to nearly 30 percent in those over 90 years. In contrast to this, the percentage of those who died in hospital

Table 4.2
Places of death in Rhineland-Palatinate, 1995

Places of death	Number	Percent
Hospital	5,393	44.1
Nursing home	1,559	12.8
Private home	4,856	39.8
Other	409	3.4
Total	12,217	

Source: Ochsmann et al. (1997).

dropped from 52 to 25 percent between those age cohorts. Dying at home, however, varied little over the different age groups.

Gender and marital status also had a significant influence on the place of death. Compared with men, because women lived longer, they less often died in hospitals or at home, but more often in nursing homes. Married or divorced people significantly more often died at home, while single persons comparatively often died in old peoples' and nursing homes.

In areas with a rural structure, people more often died in their private homes than in hospitals. In areas with an urban structure, however, it was quite the reverse: there, nursing homes played a significant part as the place of death. A high supply of hospital beds in urban areas also meant that people died in hospitals more often than at home.

Economic Data

Along with epidemiological data, economic calculations are the indispensable basis for an issue-related discussion about medical end-of-life decision making. Surveys from the United States and other countries show that the costs for health care increase in the last year of life. For Germany, reliable data only exist on inpatient hospital care; health insurance companies have scarcely any data on outpatient care (Busse et al. 1999).

The findings of an expert report commissioned by the Federal Health Ministry in 1995 show that the amount of medical services provided in the last year of life is greater for younger dying persons. Those dying at the age of 45 need about 30 times more health care than all people of the same age who do not die; dying 60-year-olds need 20 times more, 80-year-olds only 6 times more, and those over 90 need less than 5 times as much (Sachverständigenrat 1996).

Two independent factors are responsible for the high need for in-patient care compared with people of the same age who survive a serious illness: the number of people in need of inpatient care on the one hand and the average overall duration of hospitalization on the other. The percentage of those dying under 65 with at least one hospitalization is 7 to 8 times higher than the percentage for survivors of the same age. This multiple drops continuously in old age: from 5 times at age 70 and 4 times at age 80 to 3 times at age 90. In contrast to this, the average overall duration of hospitalization of those who die compared with those who survive drops continuously beyond the age of 40: from 31 times in 40-year-olds to 17 times in 60-year-olds and 6 times in 80-year-olds, to 4 times in 90-year-olds (table 4.3).

In order to determine how much in-home care was needed at the end of life, in one study family doctors documented the age, gender, situation at home, diagnosis, etc., on the first visit, the services rendered, the extent of care on each subsequent visit, and finally the time and place of death for 47 terminal patients. The frequency of physician-patient contact increased from 0.7 in the patients' tenth from last week to 2.4 in their last week of life. The family doctors mainly rendered personal care services and hardly any technical services (which because of the existing remuneration system led to insufficient remuneration of the physicians). The extent of care given by relatives rose to more than 13 hours per day in the last week of life; at that time more than 80 percent of the patients were looked after by a visiting nursing service (but only for approximately 3 hours per day). Thirty-two patients died at home, 7 in nursing homes, and 8 in hospitals after an average stay of 6 days (Busse et al. 1999).

In summary, one can say that in view of the fact that less than 50 percent of Germans die in hospitals demonstrates that dying at home deserves special interest. Without doubt, there is a great need for research both from the epidemiological and the health economics point of view.

Table 4.3
Average number of days in hospital for terminal patients and survivors

Age	Survivors		Persons in third from last year of life		Persons in second from last year of life		Persons in last year of life	
	Days		Days	Multiple	Days	Multiple	Days	Multiple
–24	0.8		9.3	11.6	11.2	14.0	24.2	29.2
25–34	0.9		13.4	14.9	12.0	13.3	28.6	30.8
35–44	1.1		13.7	12.5	22.5	20.5	34.7	31.0
45–54	1.9		11.0	5.8	15.5	8.2	39.2	21.1
55–64	2.3		6.9	3.0	12.4	5.4	40.6	17.6
65–74	3.0		9.0	3.0	12.4	4.1	36.4	12.0
75–84	4.8		8.5	1.8	11.4	2.4	31.8	6.6
85+	5.4		5.1	0.9	6.3	1.2	23.2	4.3

Source: Busse et al. (1999).

Availability of Palliative Care

In Germany there are different initiatives, institutions, and models for palliative care for seriously ill and dying persons, which can be grouped into the categories of palliative care units, inpatient hospices, day hospices, outpatient palliative care services, and outpatient hospice services.

Palliative care units are independent units affiliated with or integrated into a hospital. There is an average of eight beds and medical care is provided 24 hours a day. The treatment aims to alleviate pain and other symptoms so that the patient is able to return home. The daily costs for a palliative care unit amount to approximately $340 per bed and they are paid at 100 percent by the health insurance companies.

Hospices are, as a rule, independent institutions with independent organizational structures. They care for the most seriously ill—those with a highly advanced incurable disease and limited life expectancy. There is an average of nine beds. Some hospices are affiliated with a day hospice that offers outpatient care for patients and their relatives in order to enable patients to remain in their home setting for as long as possible. German hospices normally do not employ physicians, and medical care is mostly given by family doctors. The costs per day for inpatient care at a hospice amount to approximately $225 per bed (including medical care). These are covered by a mix of funds, consisting of reimbursements by the health and long-term care insurers, donations, and possible contributions by the patients.

Outpatient palliative care services together with general practitioners and other palliative care institutions care for seriously ill and dying patients at home. The work is focused on the supervision of pain therapy and control of symptoms. The costs per day for an outpatient palliative care service amount to $150 per patient. These costs are often not covered by health insurance companies. Therefore, most palliative care services finance themselves (in addition) by donations and third-party funding.

In contrast to outpatient palliative care services, where physicians and caregivers are experienced in palliative care work, outpatient hospice services are staffed mostly by volunteers who have no medical training. They provide personal care and conversation for the most seriously ill

Table 4.4
Development of palliative-care institutions in Germany

Year	Palliative care units and total number of beds	Hospices and total number of beds	Home-care services
1983	1 (5)	—	n.d.
1986	1 (5)	1 (53)	n.d.
1993	21 (137)	11 (165)	81
1995	26 (230)	29 (339)	198
1997	34 (299)	37 (325)	396
1999	50 (418)	64 (571)	582
2000	65 (528)	87 (771)	611

Source: Sabatowski (2000).
n.d., no data.

and dying patients and their relatives at their homes or at inpatient units. Contact with relatives frequently continues beyond the patient's death. This work is nearly exclusively financed by donations.

Compared with other European countries, palliative care units have developed relatively late and slowly in Germany. The first palliative care unit was established in 1983 at the University Hospital of Cologne; the first hospice began work in 1986 in Aachen. The crucial impetus was given in 1991 when the Federal Health Ministry began to support the establishment of palliative care units in the framework of model projects, leading to a significant increase in palliative-care units and beds (table 4.4).

In spite of great progress during the past 10 years, a sufficient supply of services for all patients needing palliative care is still not available in Germany. The need for palliative care beds, based on the experience of countries with developed palliative medical infrastructures, is estimated at 50 beds per million inhabitants. In the year 2000, however, there were only 6.4 palliative beds and 9.4 hospice beds per million inhabitants, with considerable regional differences (Müller-Busch et al. 2001). Outpatient care is also very much in need of development. On the one hand, the total number of palliative care services is impressive; on the other hand, however, of the 582 outpatient services existing as of April 1999, only 20 fulfilled the criteria of a highly qualified palliative care service

(Klaschik et al. 2000). Thus, great efforts are still necessary to achieve sufficient palliative care in Germany.

The German Debate on Medical Decisions at the End of Life

This section examines the current debate on medical decisions at the end of life. First, the current legal situation and the position of the medical professional associations are described. Second, since both emphasize the significance of the patient's will, attention is directed to the possibility of advance directives in accordance with the law in force. Finally, the relationship between theoretical discussion and clinical practice is examined.

Legal Regulations and Court Decisions

In Germany, one must distinguish among four forms of medical decisions at the end of life: active euthanasia, assisted suicide, and indirect and passive euthanasia. Legal regulations exist only for active euthanasia. For the other categories, there are only court decisions and professional ethical guidelines and recommendations by medical specialist associations.

Active euthanasia consists of deliberately shortening a life by killing the dying person. It is prohibited by criminal law, even if it is carried out on demand of the person concerned (killing on demand, § 216 criminal code). The danger of misuse and fundamental doubts ("respect for human life as such"; Landgericht Ravensburg 1987: 292) are given as reasons for the ban.

In contrast to active euthanasia, assisted suicide is not punishable in Germany. At the patient's request, the physician is allowed to put a lethal poison at his or her disposal. However, if the patient takes this poison in the doctor's presence, the physician as a guarantor is obliged to do everything possible to prevent death (Bundesgerichtshof 1984). This absurd legal situation makes assisted suicide a humanly difficult option because it forces the person administering euthanasia to leave the dying person at the end in order to escape prosecution.

So-called "indirect euthanasia" is legally admissible. This is a form of unintentional shortening of life that may occur as a side effect of the administration of high doses of analgesics. According to German courts, alleviation of pain takes precedence over a mere prolongation of life. The law is clearly against any form of "heroism of suffering" and against "imposing a duty to live," and aims to guarantee freedom from pain in accordance with the possibilities of palliative medicine (Rothärmel 2001: 724).

Most questions arise concerning passive euthanasia, which means letting the patient die by forgoing intensive care measures. In the mid-1980s, courts ruled that there was "no legal obligation for sustaining at any cost a life that is coming to an end" (Bundesgerichtshof 1984: 379), and there was no difference from the legal point of view between withholding and withdrawing (intensive care) treatment (Landgericht Ravensburg 1987). In both cases, the patient was already in the process of dying and had in the past explicitly declared herself against the intensive care measure concerned.

Matters are, however, difficult and controversial if the process of dying has not yet begun and there is no explicit declaration of the will of the patient. The Federal Court of Justice had to adjudicate such a case in 1994 (Bundesgerichtshof 1994). The regional court of Kempten had imposed a fine on the treating physician and the son, who acted as the legal guardian of a 72-year-old woman, for attempted manslaughter. On the recommendation of the physician, he and her son had agreed on terminating artificial feeding of the woman, who was severely brain injured after cardiac arrest; they expected painless death to occur after 2 to 3 weeks. The Federal Court of Justice reversed the judgment against the defendants and referred the case to the regional court for a re-hearing. As a result of this, both defendants were acquitted.

The Federal Court of Justice preceded its decision with some general guidelines. According to these, omitting life-sustaining measures may be admissible even if the process of dying has not yet begun. The presumed will of the patient is crucial. In order to establish this presumed will, past written and oral expressions by the patient, his or her religious views, additional personal values, and life expectancy in relation to the patient's age or the suffering of pain have to be taken into consideration. According to the court, if no indications for the establishment of the individual's presumed will can be found, one has to fall back on criteria that fulfill general moral concepts.

The Policy of the German Medical Association
The development initiated by the "Kempten judgment" of the Federal Court of Justice induced the German Medical Association to revise its guidelines on medical terminal care that had only been passed in 1993. In view of the social significance and explosive nature of the topic, it decided on an unusual and to-date unique procedure. In May 1997, the first draft of the new guidelines worked out by an interdisciplinary committee was presented to the public (Bundesärztekammer 1997). On the basis of the public debate, the draft was revised and again presented to the public and discussed at a conference in January 1998. The final version of the "principles on medical terminal care by the German Medical Association" was passed and published in September 1998 (Bundesärztekammer 1998).

In line with this pioneering procedure by the German Medical Association, in the principles, "paternalistic character of former guidelines" (Beleites 1998: 2366) was abolished and the patient's right to self-determination stressed. The significance and binding nature of advance directives were explicitly pointed out and terminal care was named as a task of the physician. Furthermore, it was stressed that the physician should try to find consensus with his medical and nursing staff concerning his decision making.

The differentiation between basic care and medical treatment is of fundamental importance for the principles. Basic care consists of accommodations in conditions suitable for human beings; personal care; personal hygiene; alleviating pain, respiratory distress, and nausea; as well as relieving hunger and thirst. It is indispensable and every patient is entitled to it regardless of the treatment objective. With medical treatment it is different. The physician's duty to sustain life does not exist at all costs. There are situations where diagnoses and therapies that would normally be appropriate are no longer indicated, but have to be limited. Here palliative medical care comes to the fore. The decision for this care must not—such is the demand by the German Medical Association—be dependent on economic considerations.

Most important concerning dying patients is provision of care in order to enable a dignified dying process and the alleviation of pain. Measures to prolong life may only be withheld or withdrawn in accordance with the patient's will. An intentional shortening of life by measures causing death, however, is prohibited. Assisted suicide is also rejected by the German Medical Association because of its being contradictory to medical ethos. Moreover, the patient's right to truthful disclosure is stressed.

For patients with an unfavorable prognosis or other life-threatening damage (e.g., persistent vegetative state) who are not yet dying, a change in the treatment objective and the withholding of life-sustaining measures in agreement with the patient's will may, according to the German Medical Association, only be considered if the disease is already very advanced. This restriction—which had not been included in the draft—is contradictory to the law in force. In current law, the right and the duty to treat follow from the patient's consent to treatment alone. Thus, the continuation or introduction of a life-sustaining measure against the patient's will is unlawful, regardless of the stage of the disease.

In the paragraph on the determination of the patient's will, the German Medical Association makes it clear that the patient's will takes precedence over what is useful from the medical point of view. In determining this will, a clear hierarchy of decisions must be followed. If the patient is competent, the physician will have to comply with the currently expressed will of the appropriately informed patient, even if this will does not coincide with the measures that are deemed necessary from the medical point of view. In the case of incompetent patients, the declaration of the legal representative, e.g., the parents, guardian, or authorized representative, is decisive. If there is no declaration either from the patient or from a legal representative or if it cannot be obtained in time, the physician will have to act in accordance with the patient's presumed will in the specific situation. The German Medical Association disapproves of reverting to "general moral concepts," as was suggested by the Federal Court of Justice.

The Patient's Will: The Significance of Medical Advance Directives

With the strong emphasis on the patient's will in the "Kempten judgment" of the Federal Court of Justice and in the principles on medical terminal care by the German Medical Association, the legal problems concerning medical decisions at the end of life have shifted to the determination of an incompetent patient's will. As a result of this, medical advance directives gain importance.

According to German law, the patient has three possibilities for expressing treatment wishes before a severe or fatal disease occurs: the directive for treatment known as a living will, the proxy directive as a directive for a guardian, and the durable power of attorney for health care, which offers the possibility of engaging a person of one's own choice to look after one's most personal interests.

A living will is a written or oral expression of the will of a competent person for future treatment in case of the incapability of expressing it. It contains statements on the manner and extent of medical treatment, with the option of complete rejection, but also with the possible wish for continuation of treatment or maximum treatment. The binding nature of living wills, just like the living will itself, has not yet been explicitly regulated by law. It has, however, been approved by the medical profession. Corresponding to the guidelines by the German Medical Association, the patient's will expressed in the directive is valid unless concrete indications for the patient's change of will exist (Bundesärztekammer 1998 and 1999). This is a clear rejection of the general disregard for living wills still to be found in practice that is justified by the assumption that the patient might have changed his or her mind.

The proxy directive gives the patient the opportunity to make written suggestions, if a guardianship is established by the guardianship court, as to the person who will be appointed guardian as well as the way it is to be carried out. The guardian and the physician have to follow the directive on how to carry out the guardianship as long as complying with the wishes of the patient does not go directly against his or her well-being and the guardian can be expected to comply. The guardian has to observe both the proxy directive and the living will.

In contrast to the guardian, the authorized representative is a person selected and appointed by the patient. Just like the guardian, this person is able to make decisions concerning personal matters when the patient is no longer capable of expressing his or her will. If the matters to be dealt with can be handled by an authorized representative, according to German law, the appointment of a guardian by the guardianship court is not necessary.

Until some years ago, the advantage of a durable power of attorney for health care was also that the decision of the authorized representative did not need the approval of the guardianship court. Because of this, many people signed durable powers of attorney for health care in the knowledge that a trusted person—and not the guardianship court— would make decisions on health care matters in agreement with their wishes and their well-understood interests when they were no longer capable of doing so.

This situation changed on January 1, 1999. On this day, an amendment of the guardianship law entered into force under which the authorized representative's consent also needs the approval of a judge for measures that may result in the patient's death or suffering a severe and long-lasting impairment of health. According to an interpretation of the Federal Court of Justice (1984)—which is quite controversial among jurists—the requirement of approval concerning surrogate health care decisions also applies to the termination of life-sustaining measures.

This regulation contradicts the objective of a durable power of attorney for health care. Its purpose is preventive control of the patient's representative. This control may be appropriate for a guardian appointed by the guardianship court who is unknown to the person in need of care. The authorized representative, however, is a trusted person appointed by the patient concerned. For the state to treat this representative with fundamental mistrust seems to be inappropriate, especially since the law offers the possibility of appointing a guardian to control the authorized representative if misuse of the power of attorney is suspected.

Clinical Practice

The theoretical significance of advance directives bears no relation to their actual role in clinical practice at present. Surveys on this subject show a sobering picture: of 100 mainly older people in a hospital ward, only 20 knew the term "living will" and only four had drawn up such a document. This poor knowledge is probably due to avoidance of the problem; only one quarter of the patients questioned had talked with relatives, friends, or their physician about how they would like to be treated medically and cared for in case of incompetence (Roy et al.

2002). A similar picture was revealed by a survey of 206 patients in a geronto-psychiatric ward; only 11 patients (5.4 percent) had established a living will or durable power of attorney for health care (Haupt et al. 1999), although 128 patients (62.7 percent) approved on principle of drawing up such a document.

Physicians' attitudes toward living wills, however, seem to be surprisingly positive. In a recent survey (Stolz 2002), in which approximately 1,500 physicians with their own practice from all over Germany took part, 84.5 percent of those interviewed described living wills as "helpful" and a further 14.5 percent as "partly helpful." Ninety-nine percent of the interviewees were prepared to include living wills in the patient's records. Nearly half of the general practitioners (48.3 percent) and half of the internal specialists (50.4 percent) stated that they had been guided in their decisions for treatment by a living will during the past 2 years. The frequency of the treatment decisions influenced by living wills varied between once and 40 times; the average was 3 to 4 times. The larger the number of geriatric patients that were treated in the practice, the more often living wills were taken into account.

This positive picture is put into perspective, however, when the physicians were asked about concrete decisions in concrete cases instead of general attitudes. Nearly 7 percent of the interviewed physicians would hospitalize a demented patient who had suffered a stroke with paralysis of deglutition (swallowing) and pneumonia, even if the patient had clearly declared him or herself against such a step in a valid living will. Almost half (46.7 percent) of the physicians would forgo hospitalization if this decision was supported by the guardian or authorized representative, and only 42 percent would be prepared to unreservedly follow the patient's will as set down in a living will.

This is further put into perspective by the fact that among physicians, there is considerable unawareness and uncertainty concerning the boundary between permitted passive and prohibited active euthanasia. In a survey of 1,058 physicians who participated in oncological and palliative medical continuing education in Rhineland-Palatinate from 1995 to 1999, 48.8 percent described the withdrawing of artificial respiration and 25.1 percent the termination of catecholamine administration in an intensive care patient as active euthanasia, although from the legal point of view, these measures belong to the field of passive euthanasia. Furthermore, 45.4 percent described fluid supply by tube and 30.2 percent tube feeding as indispensable basic care, while the German Medical Association wrote in its principles on medical terminal care that only the alleviation of a subjective feeling of hunger or thirst is part of basic care; supplying artificial fluid and nutrition is not (Weber et al. 2001).

Concluding Remarks

The public debate on medical end-of-life decision making in Germany was characterized by taboos and avoidance until far into the 1990s, above all for historical reasons. The fact that the term "euthanasia" was misused by the National Socialists as a guise for the eugenically motivated murder of mentally and physically disabled people not only made the discussion on medical end-of-life decision making more difficult, but was paradoxically also responsible for the delayed development of palliative care and the hospice movement in Germany (Lunshof and Simon 2000).

This has changed in the past few years. The majority of those involved in the debate have realized that historical responsibility must not lead to a suppression of present problems. The debate has become more open and diverse, but has retained its theoretical character. There is still a lack of sound empirical data for an appropriate debate on making medical decisions at the end of life.

Improvement is also necessary concerning palliative care supply facilities. Things have changed a lot in the past few years, but the situation cannot be regarded as satisfactory at all. In many parts of Germany there is a lack of beds and qualified outpatient services. Furthermore, better linking of inpatient and outpatient facilities is needed.

Last, but not least, there is a need for legal clarification concerning medical decisions at the end of life in view of the legal uncertainties that exist in practice. This especially concerns the question of the binding nature of living wills and the requirement of approval by a judge before a guardian or authorized representative can request the termination of life-sustaining measures. Moreover, the law should make it clear that neither withholding or withdrawing a life-sustaining measure at the patient's request nor the shortening of life as a side effect of a necessary medication desired by the patient constitute the offense of killing on demand.

References

Baumann, J., Bochnik, H. J., Brauneck, A. E., and Callies, R. P. 1986. *Alternativentwurf eines Gesetzes über Sterbehilfe* (AE-Sterbehilfe). Stuttgart: Thieme.

Beleites, E. 1998. Sterbebegleitung—Wegweiser für ärztliches Handeln. *Deutsches Ärzteblatt* 95 (139): A-2365–2366.

Bickel, H. 1998. Das letzte Lebensjahr: Eine Repräsentativstudie an Verstorbenen. Wohnsituation, Sterbeort und Nutzung von Versorgungsangeboten. *Zeitschrift für Gerontologie und Geriatrie* 31 (3): 193–204.

Bundesärztekammer. 1997. Entwurf der Richtlinie der Bundesärztekammer zur ärztlichen Sterbebegleitung und den Grenzen zumutbarer Behandlung. *Deutsches Ärzteblatt* 94 (20): A-1342–1344.

Bundesärztekammer. 1998. Grundsätze der Bundesärztekammer zur ärztlichen Sterbebegleitung. *Deutsches Ärzteblatt* 95 (39): A-2366–2367.

Bundesärztekammer. 1999. Handreichungen für Ärzte zum Umgang mit Patientenverfügungen. *Deutsches Ärzteblatt* 96 (43): A-2720–2721.

Bundesgerichtshof. 1984. Urteil vom 04.07.2002. BGHSt 32, 367 ff.

Bundesgerichtshof. 1994. Urteil vom 13.09.1994. BGHSt 40, 257–272.

Busse, R., Krauth, C., Wagner, H-P., Schwartz, F. W., Claes, C., and Graf von der Schulenburg, M-J. 1999. Lebensalter, Sterben und Kosten—was wissen wir über den Zusammenhang? In *Public-Health-Forschung in Deutschland*, edited by Public-Health Forschungiverbünde in der Deutschen Gesellschaft für Public Health e.V. Bern: Huber.

Federal Statistical Office Germany, http://www.destatis.de (accessed October 2002).

Haupt, M., H. Seeber, and M. Jänner, 1999. Patientenverfügungen und Bevollmächtigungen in gesundheitlichen Angelegenheiten älterer psychisch kranker Menschen. *Der Nervenarzt* 70 (3): 256–261.

Hoffmann, E., and H. Adolph. 2001. Orte des Sterbens: Eine Recherche zur Datenlage. *Informationsdienst Altersfragen* 28 (11/12): 4–5.

Klaschik, E., Nauch, F., Radbruch, L., and Sabatowski, R. 2000. Palliativmedizin: Definitionen und Grundzüge. *Internist* 41 (7): 606–611.

Landgericht Ravensburg. 1987. Urteil vom 03.12.1986, NStZ 1987, 229.

Lunshof, J., and A. Simon. 2000. Die Diskussion um Sterbehilfe und Euthanasie in Deutschland von 1945 bis in die Gegenwart. In *"Euthanasie" und die aktuelle Sterbehilfe-Debatte. Die historischen Hintergründe medizinischer Ethik*, edited by Andreas Frewer and Clemens Eickhoff. Frankfurt, New York: Campus, pp. 237–249.

Müller-Busch, H. C., I. Andres, and T. Jehser. 2001. Wie viele Palliativstationen und Hospize brauchen wir in Deutschland? *Zeitschrift für Palliativmedizin* 2 (1): 16–19.

Ochsmann, R., Slangen, K., Feith, G., Klein, D., and Seibert, A. 1997. *Sterbeorte in Rheinland-Pfalz: Zur Demographie des Todes. Beiträge zur Thanatologie,* Vol. 8. Mainz: Interdisziplinärer Arbeitskreis Thanatologie.

Rothärmel, S. 2001. Einstellung von Sondenernährung, Patientenverfügung und gerichtliche Genehmigung der Therapiebegrenzung: Zu Rechtsfragen ärztlicher Sterbehilfe. *Zentralblatt für Chirurgie* 126: 722–729.

Roy, D., Eibach, U., Röhrich, B., Nicklas-Faust, J., and Schaefer, K. 2002. Wie denken eigentlich Patienten über Patientenverfügungen? Ergebnisse einer prospektiven Studie. *Zeitschrift für Medizinische Ethik* 48: 71–83.

Sabatowski, R. 2000. Über die Entwicklung palliativmedizinischer Einrichtungen in Deutschland. *Zeitschrift für Palliativmedizin* 1 (2): 40–46.

Sachverständigenrat für die Konzertierte Aktion im Gesundheitswesen. 1996. *Gesundheitswesen in Deutschland: Kostenfaktor und Zukunftsbranche.* Vol. I: Demographie, Morbidität, Wirtschaftlichkeitsreserven. Baden-Baden: Nomos.

Stolz, K. 2002. Beurteilung von vorsorglichen Verfügungen: Was hat sich bewährt Sozial.de http://www.sozial.de (accessed April 2002).

van Oorschot, B., Dressel, G., Erdmann, B., Hausman, C., and Hildenbrand, B. 2002. "Places of death in Jena, Thüringen, in 1999." *Journal of Cancer Research and Clinical Oncology,* suppl. to Vol. 128: 158.

Weber, M., Stiehl, M., Reiter, J. and Rittner, C. 2001. Ethische Entscheidungen am Ende des Lebens—Sorgsames Abwägen der jeweiligen Situation. Ergebnisse einer Ärztebefragung in Rheinland-Pfalz. *Deutsches Ärzteblatt* 98 (48): A-3184–3188.

5

End-of-Life Decision Making in India

Sunil K. Pandya

India is the seventh largest country in the world in area. About 30 percent of the population falls below the poverty line, with a higher percentage of poor in the rural areas.

Early in the twentieth century India had birth and death rates that were both relatively high. Population growth was slow. Then, death rates fell while birth rates remained higher. As a result, population numbers have surged. On May 11, 2000, with the birth of a baby girl named Astha—"Faith" in Hindi—India's population officially hit 1 billion (Mishra 2000). The estimated population of India in October 2000 was 1,012,000,000 (Indian Society for Medical Statistics 2003). The Indian population continues to grow and is projected to become the largest of any country on earth within the next few decades.

The majority of the population lives in poverty in villages and small towns. Periodic catastrophes such as droughts, floods, famines, and epidemics drive the rural poor into the cities to eke out a living. Such migrations of large numbers with increasing frequency have imposed intolerable burdens on the infrastructure and services within the large cities, almost leading to their collapse. Huge slums house the poor in inhuman conditions. Most of those in the large cities are abjectly poor or belong to the middle class. The rich form a minority. Health services are available only to a fortunate few.

India lacks a structured health program with interconnected, efficiently functioning primary, secondary, and tertiary health centers. Public health measures are poorly implemented. We lack community services or lay health care. The concept of health visitors is almost unknown. The role played by experienced but relatively untutored women during childbirth has not been replicated in the care of the seriously ill, those with chronic diseases, or the aged. In Western countries, trained nurses with psycho-social skills working in community support teams have gained a signifi-cant degree of autonomy. This has not happened here. Nurses in India function under the dominance of the doctors. Medical insurance is in its infancy and only a minuscule segment of the population is covered by it (Gumber and Kulkarni 2000; Gupta 2002). Most patients must pay for all forms of medical treatment themselves.

India has a multiplicity of treatment regimes. These range from the allopathic system to traditional healing and home remedies. Poor vil-lagers have little access to sophisticated medical care. At best they are able to seek the help of local physicians. Since doctors trained in modern medicine are loath to practice in villages, patients must make do with the care offered by Ayurvedic (a traditional holistic system of health care in India) doctors, practitioners of homeopathy, or persons who, having served as compounders or assistants to doctors in nearby towns, have now set up practice themselves, without any formal education or certification.

Serious illness may prompt referrals to doctors in nearby towns or poorly equipped and staffed civil hospitals. A study conducted by the Indian Institute of Public Opinion showed that 88 percent of rural patients have to travel up to 8 km using inefficient and time-consuming transport to get access to medical treatment. The remaining 11 percent have to travel even farther. More than 20 percent put off buying drugs prescribed for them as far as possible in order to save money (D'Silva 2001).

Many patients with complex illnesses will succumb while in transit from their village to a doctor or to the civil hospital. A small number may reach a government or municipal hospital in a large city. When attached to medical colleges, these hospitals are well equipped and staffed, although recently cracks are appearing even in these edifices, and we see weakening standards. Sophisticated therapy, including a stay in intensive care units and major operations such as those on the heart and brain, is available here. The government or municipal corpo-ration absorbs most of the costs. Even so, the patient's family can incur significant expense for travel to and from the hospital and a stay in the big city, where costs are much higher than those in the village. The custom of having large numbers of relatives accompany each seriously ill person further increases the spending. Moreover, often they must buy drugs and other necessary items because these are out of stock at the hospital.

Garg (1998) concluded his study on costs in health care in India with the following findings. Both government and private expenditures are higher for higher income quintiles and for people living in urban areas and working in an organized sector. The organized sector, as the name implies, has official organization, such as a registered office or factory. This is in contrast to individuals or groups who function by themselves with no backing, support, or even regular location. The itinerant barber, laborer, or day hire are examples. On the other hand, people in the lower income quintile and in rural areas bear a higher burden of health expenditures as a proportion of their income. Delivery of health care is also biased in favor of urban areas.

Difficulties in Obtaining Data in India

While trying to obtain data on the costs of dying and death in India, it soon became obvious that surveys were impossible in a country where there is no information even on expenditures on medical care or causes of death. Gupta highlights one aspect of such difficulties in collecting data: "Most individuals in the low-income households actually did not either recall or know at all how much was spent on these items (expenditure on health care), which resulted from visits to a doctor" (2002: 2795). Only a small proportion of our population receives medical attention at the time of death.

Calculating the cost of dying in the large cities is also complex. The causes of death vary by age and sex. There are wide variations in medical expenditure at the time of death because of the duration and kind of treatment received for terminal illnesses. Public health and health economics are given low priorities in Indian universities, thus it is not surprising that there are no studies on such topics in India.

The Essence of Indian Philosophy on Death

India has fostered many cultures. The following teachings are a sample from the ancient Indian classics. This philosophy permeates the psyche of the vast majority of Indians, heirs to the Hindu, Buddhist, Jain, Sikh, and other allied cultures.

The infinite is bliss. There is no bliss in anything finite.
He who sees this does not see death, nor illness, nor pain. (*Khandogya Upanishad*; 23rd and 26th Khanda)

This body is mortal and always held by death. It is the abode of that Self which is immortal and without body. When in the body (by thinking this body is I and I am this body) the Self is held by pleasure and pain. So long as he is in the body, he cannot get free from pleasure and pain. But when he is free of the body (when he knows himself different from the body), then neither pleasure nor pain touches him. (*Khandogya Upanishad*; Eighth Prapathaka, 12th Khanda)

He who knows at the same time both the cause and the destruction (the perishable body), overcomes death by destruction (the perishable body), and obtains immortality through (knowledge of) the true cause. (*Isa Upanishad*)

One of the most important words in the ancient philosophy of the Brahmans is Âtman, nom. sing. Âtmâ. It is rendered in our dictionaries by "breath, soul, the principle of life and sensation, the individual soul, the self, the abstract individual, self, one's self, the reflexive pronoun, the natural temperament -or disposition, essence, nature, character, peculiarity, the person or the whole body, the body, the understanding, intellect, the mind, the faculty of thought and reason, the thinking faculty, the highest principle of life, Brahma, the supreme deity or soul of the universe, care, effort, pains, firmness, the Sun, fire, wind, air, a son." (Muller 1879: xxviii, Vol. 1, part 1)

Desireless, wise, immortal, self-existent, full of bliss, lacking in nothing, is the one who knows the wise, unaging, youthful Âtman: he fears not death! (Atharva Veda X, 8, 446)

Nachiketas enters into the abode of Yama Vaivasvata. Granted three boons by Yama, Nachiketas addresses him thus: "In the heaven-world there is no fear; thou art not there, O Death, and no one is afraid on account of old age. Leaving behind both hunger and thirst, and out of the reach of sorrow, all rejoice in the world of heaven."

In response, after considerable reluctance, Yama explains: "The good is one thing, the pleasant another; these two, having different objects, chain a man. It is well with him who clings to the good; he who chooses the pleasant, misses his end. The good and the pleasant approach man: the wise goes round about them and distinguishes them. Yea, the wise prefers the good to the pleasant, but the fool chooses the pleasant through greed and avarice."

"The knowing Self is not born, it dies not; it sprang from nothing, nothing sprang from it. The Ancient is unborn, eternal, everlasting; he is not killed, though the body is killed."

"A man who is free from desires and free from grief, sees the majesty of the Self by the grace of the Creator. The wise who knows the Self as bodiless within the bodies, as unchanging among changing things, as great and omnipresent, does never grieve."

"He who has perceived that which is without sound, without touch, without form, without decay, without taste, eternal, without smell, without beginning, without end, beyond the Great, and unchangeable, is freed from the jaws of death."

"Having understood that the senses are distinct (from the Âtman), and that their rising and setting (their waking and sleeping) belongs to them in their distinct existence (and not to the Âtman), a wise man grieves no more."

"When all desires that dwell in his heart cease, then the mortal becomes immortal, and obtains Brahman."

When all the ties of the heart are severed here on earth, then the mortal becomes immortal." (Nachiketa's Experiences with Yama, the Lord of Death in the *Katha Upanishad*)

These and other traditional teachings can be summed up by the following points:

1. Time (*kala*) is not considered rectilinear but cyclical (Filippi 1996).

2. All that is material—including the human body, mind, and intellect—is of little consequence. Those who remain attached to material objects are condemned to the cycle of birth—death—rebirth.

3. The ultimate goal of the enlightened is freedom from rebirth after death through the attainment of union with the Brahman (God or the universal spirit). Toward this goal, freedom from desire has to be consciously achieved. Such an individual, knowing that the Âtman (the essence of the person) is distinct from the body, is not grieved by death.

4. For the enlightened individual, death is welcome as the means by which freedom from the cycle of rebirth can be achieved.

Some Medically Relevant Consequences of Indian Philosophy

Belief in the cycle of rebirth robs death of much of its terror, although the loss of a loved one continues to cause grief. Several Indian faiths—notably Jainism—honor individuals in good health and full possession of their senses who, having lived full lives, decide to die. Such an individual literally starves to death. The medical profession is in no way involved in the decision or its implementation. Such a person is said not to die but to relinquish his body. The community honors this intent and practice and reveres the memory of persons who, in its opinion, are fortunate enough to achieve such good deaths. Euthanasia has a different connotation here.

The prolongation of the process of dying when life has lost its meaning is anathema to the Indian psyche. The use of sense-deadening drugs or surgery in terminally ill individuals is frowned upon. This follows the belief that the Âtman can leave the body at different levels. When it leaves the body through the top of the head, the person is freed from the cycle of rebirth. To ensure this, the dying person must retain the highest degree of awareness. When consciousness is clouded, the soul leaves the body at inferior levels, leading to rebirth.

There is a general acceptance of the fact that the human remains after death are no longer the beloved relative or friend. This explains why a son will break open the skull of his dead father at the funeral pyre with great serenity to facilitate the exit of the last psychic energy (Filippi 1996).

Since death implies liberation of the Âtman from the mortal shell that housed it, the corpse is inconsequential. The removal of organs from a corpse to benefit sick individuals has met with rapid general approval from community leaders and religious heads. An example of such philosophy in action is provided in the last will of Professor Prabodh Chandra Sen who was a renowned scholar of Bengali rhythmics and an author of many books on Indian history and Rabindranath Tagore. A few hours before he died at the age of 89, he stated that instead of having his corpse burned, he would like to have it given to some medical institution so that it could be utilized as needed by patients or students.

In times past, Indian philosophy provided a coping mechanism for the bereaved. However, Western influences in towns and cities have cut the younger generation adrift from their cultural moorings, with consequent difficulties in coming to terms with suffering and death.

Sick people turn first to their families for help and here we are fortunate. There is a deep sense of belonging within families and communities. This is especially evident in villages and small towns and ensures care of the mentally handicapped, infirm, and aged at all times. Any crisis—and serious illness is one such—immediately results in an outpouring of assistance in various forms from other members of the family and from the community.

Until a few decades ago, most deaths occurred at home. The family cared for the sick person, doing all that was possible and calling in the physician for medical advice. This practice continues in villages and small towns, especially when the illness is prolonged or degenerative.

This cohesive, beneficial social force is weakening in metropolitan cities where joint families have given way to nuclear households or single-parent homes. One obvious consequence is the development of homes for the aged. It is interesting that it is the financially well-off families that tend to deposit their elders in such homes. The wide dispersal of family members within the country and abroad has resulted in early hospitalization because there is no one at home to look after the seriously ill person. Many deaths now occur in hospitals or nursing homes.

Economic Factors: Few Are Blessed with a Swift, Short, Terminal Illness

Ideal care—as would be deemed mandatory in Western countries—is available only to those who can afford to travel and stay in private clinics or centers in smaller towns or in the large metropolitan public or private hospitals. Costs in private clinics and hospitals may be tenfold or more than those in the public centers.

Members of the upper middle class also are often hard put to cope with serious illnesses. It is not uncommon for those working in intensive care units (ICUs) in major private hospitals to be asked by anxious relatives of patients whose survival is in question: "How long will this patient need to stay in the ICU? We are now running out of funds." The situation is especially pathetic when the patient is beyond help but cannot yet be declared dead. The query, prompted by huge bills in the face of a hopeless situation, is now tinged with desperation: "When do you think all this will end?" One can sense a wish—suppressed only because of societal pressures—to ask, "Can you not stop treatment?" After the death of the patient, many families have lamented the financially crippling decision to bring their relative to the ICU.

The increasing resort to ICUs and the use of the very expensive technologies in it by doctors treating seriously ill patients is causing a dilemma in Indian society. While the role of such units in saving life is not denied, the costs are prompting questions about the criteria for placing patients in them and whether, under certain circumstances, such treatment should not be withheld or withdrawn. The latter proposition, of course, spawns a host of medicolegal issues that are as yet unresolved. It is simpler not to hook up a patient to a ventilator than it is to disconnect the machine. Likewise, it is easier not to start a dopamine drip than to discontinue it. Only the wealthy can face the costs of treating serious illness with some degree of equanimity.

Medical Factors

In India, as elsewhere, there has been an improvement in life expectancy and a gradual shift from infectious causes of death (which remain important) to those related to cancer and degenerative diseases. AIDS poses a worsening problem. The process of dying has been prolonged by chronic diseases such as AIDS and tuberculosis, as well as those related to old age. This in turn means a greater expenditure of time, energy, and funds by other members of the family. Given the general poverty, these diseases have become a disabling burden to most families.

Malnutrition and anemia in the poor worsen their outlook when they are stricken by serious illness and render them vulnerable to further ravages by chronic diseases such as tuberculosis because of their inability to complete a prescribed therapy or attend follow-up clinics. What might be curable for those with sufficient resources proves fatal in the poor.

Age by itself plays a small role in decision making in the treatment of terminal illness. Indian culture fosters respect for the aged. There is a deep sense of obligation toward parents and elders. Duty demands that everything possible be done for them at all times. A gradual shift away from this approach is noticeable in metropolitan centers. Terminal illness in the aged imposes an intolerable financial burden on nuclear middle-class and poorer families. When the younger members of both sexes of such families have to work to earn the livelihood of the family, there is often no one to attend to the chronically ill. This recently has led to the development of agencies that care for such patients. Cultural constraints impose difficulties when the younger generation has to consider placing an ill parent into such an institution. The fear of "What will others say?" plays a major role, inhibiting such a move.

The terminally ill infant or child wrings the minds and hearts of all. The search for any means that will help often leads to great expense and distress. When modern medicine fails, resort to Ayurveda, homeopathy, and other alternative systems is common. It is only when the approach of death is obvious that resignation sets in.

Epidemics (the most recent of which is that caused by AIDS) find the country and its people poorly prepared. Panic and hysteria overtake injunctions that stem from traditional Indian philosophy. Ostracization replaces care. Pain and suffering do not evoke sympathy or the means for alleviating them. Patients are left unattended by relatives, friends, and members of the medical profession. Death is seen as nature's way of ridding the family and society of an unwelcome burden.

End-stage renal disease is an excellent example. The number of patients with such disease is huge and increases annually. The cost of treatment in each patient is very high whether we consider periodic dialysis or an organ transplant and recurring costs thereafter. Few can afford these costs. Desperation often forces families to choose organ transplantation, impoverishing them in the process. Other problems abound. Organs are not easily available and this has resulted in the creation of a black market where organs are sold and bought or even stolen. Despite public knowledge of widespread malpractice, there has been little effective corrective action either by organizations of medical professionals or the authorities. Ineffective or corrupt monitoring agencies have ensured that those making a quick profit remain unhindered while the patients and their families get cheated.

Pain Management and Palliative Care

There are a few centers in India that offer palliative care as provided in hospices abroad. These centers have been established by public-spirited persons: grants, donations, and personal contributions by the founders form the principal sources of funds. Volunteers help the small number of paid employees. The work done at a representative center, the Calicut Pain and Palliative Care Clinic, is described here as an illustration. The following information was provided by the clinic on September 2, 2002:

Number of new patients treated each year up to December 31, 2001.

1994: 387

1995: 690

1996: 1,475
1997: 1,582
1998: 1,882
1999: 2,205
2000: 1,744
2001: 2,060

On average, each patient spent Rs. 1,000 to 1,500 (US$20 to $30) per month for medicine. Poor patients (80 percent of the total) were given all medicine free of cost. Patients belonging to the middle and upper class (20 percent) were asked to buy medicine other than morphine (which is not available on sale) from the pharmacies. The center does not collect a fee for any of its services.

In many Indian centers, until recently, opioids such as morphine were not available for pain relief because of regulations to prevent their misuse and diversion. Studies on 1,723 patients who were being treated for pain with oral morphine on an outpatient home-care basis over 2 years did not identify any instances of misuse or diversion. It was concluded that oral morphine can be dispensed safely to patients for use at home. On the basis of this study, the experts at Calicut recommended that palliative care programs make the concerned government authorities aware of the medical need for opioids and communicate with local news media to increase awareness of palliative care and the use of these analgesics. Thanks to such pioneering efforts, regulatory barriers that had interrupted the availability of morphine and its use in pain relief in India have now been overcome.

Most centers offering palliative care are affiliated with institutions possessing high technology. The latter, often in the public sector, look after persons in need of such technology at relatively low cost. When a patient is terminally ill, palliative care centers take over the management completely and do their best to ensure comfort, the presence of dear ones, and a smooth passage from life to death. Toward this end, they possess the tools needed for continuous intravenous infusions of morphine and other similar drugs, the care of wounds, and minor surgery.

Experience thus far suggests that palliative care centers play an important role, but that their patterns and practices need considerable modification from those adopted in Western countries to ensure that they attract patients and are able to serve them amid abject poverty. It must be emphasized that the number of palliative care centers in India is very small and can cater to only a very small segment of the vast numbers actually in need of such attention.

Proportion of Patients Dying in Intensive Care Units, Hospitals, Hospices or Homes

We do not have reliable figures on place of death, but it is safe to say that in villages, a majority of patients die at home or in nearby clinics. Few reach a major hospital or intensive care unit. In the larger towns and cities, patients from the middle and upper classes seek treatment in intensive care units in nursing homes and hospitals, the rich preferring the large private hospitals to those run by the government or municipal corporations. A significant proportion of these patients die in hospitals. Of these, the number dying in intensive care units forms a small proportion simply because the number of intensive care beds is limited and the costs are very high. A decision to transfer a patient into an intensive care unit is usually made by the doctors, with the relatives of the patient docilely concurring.

The concept of hospice has taken root, but their number is still very small. The number of beds in hospices forms an almost insignificant fraction of all hospital beds in any region. As a consequence, there is usually a waiting list for admittance in hospices, and the number of deaths in them is small.

Cutoff Points for Aggressive Care

As yet, there is no national consensus on cutoff points. Death is, of course, a common end point, but the criteria for the diagnosis of death may vary from those for brain death (as defined by law) to the conventional permanent cessation of breathing and the heartbeat. Even when brain death is diagnosed, many centers balk at shutting off the ventilator or disconnecting all other supports when no organs are to be harvested. This reluctance follows an anomaly in the Transplantation of Human

Organs Act of 1994, passed by the Parliament of India (Kabra 1996). The act appears to define brain death only for the purposes of removal of organs for transplantation. This presumption has been strengthened by the recent notification by the Medical Council of India (equivalent to the General Medical Council in the United Kingdom), where we find the following statement in the section on euthanasia:

6.7 Euthanasia: Practicing euthanasia shall constitute unethical conduct. However on specific occasion, the question of withdrawing supporting devices to sustain cardio-pulmonary function even after brain death, shall be decided only by a team of doctors and not merely by the treating physician alone. A team of doctors shall declare withdrawal of the support system. Such team shall consist of the doctor in charge of the patient, Chief Medical Officer/Medical Officer in charge of the hospital and a doctor nominated by the in-charge of the hospital from the hospital staff or in accordance with the provisions of the Transplantation of Human Organs Act, 1994. (Medical Council of India 2002)

Such confusing statements from officious agencies have stymied those doctors wishing to withdraw all support measures once brain-death has been diagnosed. Eminent Indian jurists conclude that were a case of withdrawal of support from a brain-dead person ever to come to trial, the doctor and clinic would be exonerated. However, fear of legal action against clinician and hospital make it prudent to await conventionally defined death before certifying it and stopping all therapy. In the process, intensive care beds remain occupied, much-needed ventilators remain "in use," and very expensive care is wasted on dead persons. Care can, of course, be withdrawn on the express command of the legal heir of the brain-dead person, but such orders are rare. The heir, like the doctor, fears reprisals, this time from other relatives who may attribute ulterior motives.

Who Decides?

Decisions on all matters pertaining to treatment or its cessation are intensely personal. The head of the family is often the final authority. Males usually dominate females and it is not uncommon for the husband to make decisions on matters of life and death pertaining to his wife or daughters without even consulting them. The lack of universal health insurance or care under the aegis of a social security blanket ensures that government agencies play no role.

The medical community can and does influence individuals and families by providing information, guidance, and, at times, paternalistic advice. Individuals and families continue to repose trust in the medical attendants and tend to follow their recommendations. Ethics committees are either nonexistent or in very primitive stages in all but a handful of medical institutions in India. They have yet to play any significant role in influencing decisions on the mode of death.

The law in India does not as yet recognize advance directives. As a consequence, few persons offer such directives. The Society for the Right to Die and other similar agencies are striving to promote consciousness on the subject, but have yet to make any dent in existing practice. The microscopic minority carrying advance directive cards—commonly refusing intensive care and heroic measures at resuscitation under specified circumstances—does so on the basis of their indoctrination while living abroad. The doctor encountering such a card does take cognizance, but action remains firmly based on what the law permits.

The law in India does not permit euthanasia or suicide. The decision by some aged Jain seers to starve themselves to death is technically illegal but has been accepted by society. The growing plea for a right to die when life has become a burden because of irreversible and progressive fatal disease has led to discussions on these subjects with increasing frequency in medical and social science institutions and under the aegis of other bodies including medical associations and institutes of social science. As yet, the consensus is against the willful termination of life by doctors under any circumstances.

Estimated Costs of Dying

It is very difficult to arrive at the costs of dying in India because of the following reasons:

- In India there is a lack of information even on the causes of death.
- Only a small proportion of the population receives medical attention for a fatal illness.
- A calculation of the cost of dying is complex because causes of death vary by age, sex, and location (village; small town or metropolis; public or private hospital). There are also differences because of the duration of

treatment received for the ailment (or ailments, in case of deaths due to multiple causes) that has resulted in death.

Verma and Srivastava (1990) conducted a field study aimed at measuring the personal cost of illness from five major water-related diseases in a rural area of Uttar Pradesh in 1981–1982. The diseases included in the study were enteric fever, acute diarrhea-related diseases, infective hepatitis, conjunctivitis, and scabies. The measurement of the cost of illness included information on losses in productivity and treatment costs. The aggregate annual costs per person of illnesses that were due to the above five diseases ranged between Rs. 221 (US$16) and Rs. 248 (US$18) in the 2 years.

Rajeswari et al. (1999) studied the socioeconomic impact of tuberculosis on patients and their families and the costs incurred by patients in rural and urban areas. The study population consisted of 304 patients (government health care, 202; nongovernmental organization, 77; private practitioner, 25), 120 of whom were females. The mean direct cost was Rs. 2052/-, indirect was Rs. 3934/-, and the total cost was Rs. 5986/- (US$171). The mean number of workdays lost was 83 and mean debts totaled Rs. 2079/-. Both rural and urban female patients faced rejection by their families (15 percent). Eleven percent of schoolchildren discontinued their studies; an additional 8 percent took up employment to support their family. The authors concluded that the total costs, and particularly indirect costs due to tuberculosis, were relatively high. The average period of loss of wages was 3 months. The caregiving activities of female patients decreased significantly and a fifth of schoolchildren discontinued their studies.

Studies such as this permit a glimpse into the costs of serious illnesses and, indirectly, of death. Neha Madhiwala provided the author with details from a study by the Center for Education, Health and Allied Technology (CEHAT) in Nashik district in Maharashtra (personal communication, 2002). Fieldwork was conducted in 1996 and covered nearly 1,200 households in Igatpuri taluka (a rural area) and Nashik City. The study focused on utilization of health care and expenditures and sources of financing for illnesses in the previous month, and maternity events and deaths in the previous year for all members of the household. The data are as yet unpublished, but they give some idea about the financial burden put on households by death and the sources of financing sought by households of different socioeconomic classes (table 5.1).

These figures can be taken as representative of most parts of India. Few persons possess insurance coverage. The bottom two rows in the table clearly show the most poignant aspect of illness and death among the poor. Already in debt, the poor sink further through supplementary borrowing and sell their meager assets.

It is difficult to comment on the proportion of health care costs expended in the last 3 to 6 months of life, but it would be fair to say that in a chronic illness such as cancer that leads to death, the cost is considerable. As noted earlier, a deep sense of duty drives the family to seek every possible avenue of cure. Considerable sums are spent on Ayurvedic, homeopathic, and other alternative forms of medicine, often against the advice of the physician who has diagnosed the fatal illness on sound scientific grounds. It is not uncommon to see poor families travel considerable distances and at great cost on hearsay evidence of a miraculous cure. The sums spent in modern intensive care units, too, are progressively rising as more and more families turn to them in an attempt at curing a loved one. The sensitive clinician is often horrified by the expenses incurred in "treating" a patient with advanced cancer and general system failure at the insistence of a family that can ill afford such costs.

Some Tentative Conclusions

Indian philosophy makes the acceptance of death easier than in Western countries. Support from other members of the family and friends eases the lot of the relatives of the dying patient. Most deaths in the young follow acute illness or accidents, while the aged succumb to chronic, crippling, or debilitating illnesses, or acute catastrophe such as a stroke or myocardial infarction.

The spread of diseases such as AIDS has wrought further havoc within an already substandard system of health care. Only a minority of the population is covered by medical insurance or has access to medical care of high quality. The poor die at home or in ill-equipped and poorly

Table 5.1
Sources of financing for death by socioeconomic class

Source	Nonworker, casual workers	Formal sector/ unskilled and semiskilled workers	Formal sector skilled/service sector worker	Professionals, and business
Own income	4.2	17.4	78.8	36.6
Insurance or employer	0	0	0	0
Credit from third party	0	3.3	0	0
Loans from relatives	74.8	17.0	17.4	31.7
Debt	10.6	16.0	2.6	31.7
Sale of assets or household goods	10.4	46.4	1.3	

staffed clinics. Few can reach intensive care units in tertiary medical centers.

Aging persons have traditionally been respected and carefully attended to up to their death, irrespective of their gender. Recent trends mirror Western practices as nuclear families find themselves unable to care for their crippled or demented elders. We are beginning to see the development of centers for the aged where such persons can be cared for at a cost. Such care falls far short of that given by devoted family members.

Increasing longevity is associated with a greater need for medical and paramedical care. Widespread poverty, the absence of specific geriatric care, very limited facilities for rehabilitation after injury or disease, and falling standards at public sector medical establishments make it difficult for the elderly to lead meaningful lives. It is not uncommon to hear an aged person lament, "I wish God will soon take me away from this world."

Palliative care centers are gradually gaining acceptance. Western models need modification to ensure acceptance and provide care to those most in need. At present they are too few to cater to more than a very small percentage of patients. Most of these centers are philanthropic, funded by donations, and offer their services free of cost.

Euthanasia by members of the medical profession remains illegal. There is little debate thus far on the right to die. The Society for the Right to Die in Mumbai has few members and desultory proceedings, notwithstanding the efforts by its founders.

Finally, there is a great need to inculcate medical students and practitioners with the principles of medical ethics and to create an effective mechanism for ensuring that all care of the sick meets the highest ethical standards.

Acknowledgments

Many persons have helped in this study. I am especially grateful to those who obtained hard-to-get data from a wide variety of sources. In alphabetical order they are Dr. Amar Jesani, Mumbai; Mr. Pranay Lal and Sarita, Health and Environment Unit, Center for Science and Environment, New Delhi; Ms. Gayatri Nayak, *The Economic Times*, Mumbai;

Dr. A. M. Pai; Dr. Sanjay Pai, Manipal Hospital, Bangalore; Dr. M. R. Rajagopal, Pain and Palliative Care Clinic, Medical College, Calicut; Mr. Kishore S. Rao; and Ms. Sandhya Srinivasan, Mumbai. I also wish to thank Dr. Robert Blank for his editing of the manuscript.

References

D'Silva, J. 2001. "Good Healthcare Is a Very Long Walk for Most Villages." *Economic Times*, January 29.

Garg, C. C. 1998. Equity of Health Care Sector Financing and Delivery in India. http://www.hsph.harvard.edu/takemi/rp144.pdf (accessed 21 March 2004).

Gumber, A., and V. Kulkarni 2000. "Health Insurance for Informal Sector." *Economic and Political Weekly* 35 (40): 3607–3613, September 30.

Gupta, I. 2002. "Private Health Insurance and Health Costs. Results from a Delhi Study." *Economic and Political Weekly:* EPW special article 37 (27): 2795–2802, July 6.

Indian Society for Medical Statistics. 2003. http://icmr.nic.in/isms/isms.htm (accessed 21 March 2004).

Kabra, S. G. 1996. *Laws in Practice of Medicine.* Jaipur: Rajasthan Voluntary Health Association.

Medical Council of India. 2002. MCI notification of April 6, 2002, the Indian Medical Council (professional conduct, etiquette, and ethics) Regulations, 2002. Published in Part III, Section 4 of the *Gazette of India*, April 6.

Mishra, N. 2000. "One More. India's Population Tops 1 Billion." May 11 http://abcnews.go.com/sections/world/DailyNews/indiababy000511.html (accessed June 2001).

Muller, F. M., ed. and trans. 1879/1900. *The Upanishads*, Vol. 15, Parts 1 and 2. The Sacred Books of the East. Oxford: Oxford University Press. Reprinted by Motilal Banarsidass, Delhi, 1975.

Rajeswari, R., R. Balasubramanian, M. Muniyandi, S. Geetharamani, X. Thresa, and P. Venkatesan. 1999. "Socio-economic Impact of Tuberculosis on Patients and Family in India." *International Journal of Tuberculosis and Lung Diseases* 10: 869–877.

Verma, B. L., and R. N. Srivastava. 1990. "Measurement of the Personal Cost of Illness Due to Some Major Water-related Diseases in an Indian Rural Population." *International Journal of Epidemiology* 19: 169–176.

6

End-of-Life Decision Making in Israel

Tali Amidror and Frank J. Leavitt

The mysteries are for God, and the revealed things are for us and for our children forever, to do all the words of this Torah.
—Deuteronomy XXIX, 28

Decisions about the end of life must always take place in a context of ignorance. No matter what we decide, we must always be conscious of the gnawing recognition that we do not have the slightest idea of what happens to us after death. Maybe there is an afterlife, and maybe there is only annihilation and emptiness. And if there is an afterlife, what can it possibly be like? Perhaps there is eternal suffering far exceeding that of the most tormented terminal patient. Or perhaps a paradise awaits us, in which we will finally learn the deep truths of God and the angels, and the secrets of the meaning of life will finally be revealed. Or maybe things are more complicated, and this life is only one of many thousands of lives that we must live in order to repair, improve, and refine our souls, as is taught in the doctrines of reincarnation of mystical kabalistic Judaism and in Hinduism. And maybe in between each life and the next, we get a kind of debriefing, in which we receive an explanation of what it has all been about. And maybe we don't get any explanation ever. And if we do get reincarnated, maybe it is always as human beings. Or maybe we sometimes become animals or plants or micro-organisms or rocks. Or maybe there will be no individual identity at all, because our minds are really only part of the infinite intellect of God, as Spinoza taught in his philosophy. The speculative possibilities are endless. All we can say if we are honest is that we have no idea what is true, if indeed any of them is true at all.

Dogmatic people "know" with absolute certainty what life and death are all about. The atheistic materialist "knows" that there is no God and no afterlife. The existentialist version of atheism "knows" that there is therefore no meaning to life except for the meaning that we create for ourselves. And some religious people "know" how to ensure for themselves an eternal Garden of Eden with infinite culinary and sexual pleasures.

Judaism tends to teach more humility. Although we affirm in general terms the existence of God and the revival of the dead, we hasten to add that we do not know very much, if anything at all, about these things. One of the central messages of Maimonides' *Guide for the Perplexed* is that we really cannot know anything about God.

In spite of all the emphasis that bioethics puts on autonomy and informed consent, it is impossible to make an informed decision to enter a situation—like death—about which we can know nothing. Not only are we ignorant about the meaning of our lives with respect to worlds afterward and a future existence, we cannot know very much about the meanings of our actions for the lives of other people. Nor can we be sure about what our lives mean to ourselves. People often change their minds radically about their religious or philosophical beliefs or choice of mate or career. A suffering patient who has decided that all he or she wants is to die as soon as possible can suddenly start to want to live at least long enough to attend a grandchild's wedding.

Nor can bystanders, family, or health professionals know anything about the meaning of a few remaining minutes of life, even for a miserable and depressed patient whose "quality of life" is nearly nonexistent by any accepted quantitative scale. Perhaps after an unreflective life devoted only to material success and pleasure, the patient is now for the first time reflecting on what it was all about, regretting injury done to others and taking consolation in some good deeds. Perhaps deep within the mind of a patient whose life appears worthless to any objective outside observer, those few moments are the first and only time when the patient has found meaning in life. Because of all the unknowns in end-of-life decision making, and because of the humility and nondogmatism that secular as well as religious Jews seem to have absorbed, it is not surprising that Israel has few laws and little consensus on these matters.

It is generally thought that in Israel the limitation of treatment for terminal patients consists of refraining from starting treatment, rather than disconnecting patients from life-support systems (Eidelman 1998), but Israeli medical practice with respect to terminal patients has not yet been sufficiently researched. From all the reports on this subject, it seems almost certain that no uniform policy exists. With no explicit law, and not even any obligatory unwritten rule, an unusual situation has come about. Today, the approach to terminal patients may differ from one medical center to another, from one ward to another within the same medical center, and sometimes from one professional to another within the same ward.

The authors of this chapter are divided on whether this lack of uniformity is a healthy or an unhealthy phenomenon. On the one hand, it can be pointed out that the lack of a clear approach in contemporary Israel causes difficulties for patients and for medical staff. The patients and their families do not know their rights. At the same time, the staff is likely to hesitate to respect the desires of the patient for fear of being brought to court on a charge of causing death. On the other hand, in a realm where the truth is a mystery, perhaps pluralism is the only reasonable solution.

In this chapter we discuss the question of refusal of treatment and coercive treatment in Halacha (Jewish Law) and in the quite unclear Patients' Rights Law of 1996, the ethical status of disconnecting life-support systems, the determination of the moment of death, euthanasia, discontinuing futile treatment, neonate intensive care, and nursing care.

Refusal of Treatment and Coercive Treatment in Israeli Religious and Secular Law

Although Israel is known as the Jewish state, and evidence of the preservation of Jewish tradition can be seen everywhere, it is not clear how much rabbinical opinion is really listened to in medical decision making. In a religious hospital, such as Sharey Tzedek in Jerusalem, rabbis may have substantial authority, but in a large, pluralistic hospital, such as Soroka Medical Centre in Beer Sheva, the role of rabbis may not consist in much more than supervision of the kosher preparation (*kashrut*) of the patients' food. On the other hand, although religious experts have little formal role in medical decision making, many of them are quite well informed about current medical developments, and participate together with medical professionals, bioethicists, and lawyers in discussions, seminars, and committees. Indeed, some of the chief experts in religious medical law, like Steinberg and Halperin, are also distinguished doctors.

Rabbinical experts have, moreover, given many decisions that are not very different from the opinions of secular bioethicists, although their reasons may be different. For example, while the right of a patient to refuse treatment may be defended in international bioethics on grounds of autonomy, rabbis have defended it for other reasons. Rabbi Shlomo Goren, former Chief Rabbi of Israel, defended it on the grounds that the great medieval rabbi, Nachmanides (Ramban) recognized the right of a patient to refuse a doctor's care and to turn to a prophet instead (Goren 1991). Rabbi Shilo Rafael, late head of a Jerusalem rabbinical court, defended this right on the grounds that although it may be the case that a patient *ought* to accept medical care, today, when there is no king in Israel, nobody has the right to force people to do what religion says they ought to do (Rafael 1992).

As for Israeli secular law, Section 13 of the Patients' Rights Law states that medical treatment will not be given to a patient unless the patient has given informed consent. However, it is not clear whether the patient has a right to refuse life-sustaining treatment. The status of advance directives is still unclear, as is the role of a surrogate. The Patients' Rights Law gives the hospital ethics committee the authority to decide if the treatment will improve the patient's condition, and to authorize such treatment even against the patient's will, if it is to be expected that the treatment will significantly improve the patient's medical condition, and if there are grounds to believe that the patient will later give retroactive consent. But it is not clear whether the committee has a right to impose treatment if a significant improvement is not foreseen. Israeli health professionals, bioethicists, lawyers, and the public are keenly aware of the need for more clarity, and work is well under way toward preparing new legislation, with proposals having been written by Dr. Carmel Shalev and Attorney Galia Hildesheimer, and by a distinguished committee chaired by Prof. Avraham Steinberg (Shalev and Hildesheimer 2001; Public Committee on the Dying Patient 2002). With the formation of the new National Unity government in February 2003, however, a new minister of health took office and proposed legislation will probably have to be reexamined. Thus, the situation is once again unclear.

Nor have the hospital ethics committees, which were mandated by the law, been a total success. Although they are legally required, a number of hospitals still do not have them, 6 years after the passage of the law. Where the committees do exist, physicians often do not bother to turn to them with ethical questions (Wenger et al. 2002). Physicians are theoretically required to turn to the ethics committee for permission to withhold medical information from patients, and for permission for coercive treatment in nonemergency situations. But if all physicians were to consult the hospital ethics committee whenever they are required to, it is doubtful that the committee would have the time to deal with all the questions.

The concept of "withholding medical information from the patient" is not very well defined. A physician who is aware of the law recently told us about the case of a patient who, in the doctor's opinion, would be endangered by knowing the truth about his condition. However, the doctor had not yet felt a need to consult the ethics committee because, as he remarked: "I have not yet concealed the truth from the patient."

Not only are the meaning of life, and the passage from life to death, mysterious, each case can be deeply different from all others. So how can we aim at uniformity of decisions? It will be sufficient if clear procedures are established, outlining the respective roles of physicians, nurses, ward social workers, patients and their families, and perhaps ethics committees in decision making. We have heard of a case in which a young registrar, alone in the ward at night, made a do-not-resuscitate (DNR) decision on his own. However, the matter of the ending of life is too profound and complex to allow even the most distinguished physician to make such decisions alone. It must be a team decision, made in the ward meeting and involving the nurses and social workers, with the patient and family considered as members of the team. The specific decisions will probably continue to vary from hospital to hospital, from ward to ward, and from patient to patient.

Disconnecting Life Support

Although active euthanasia, in the sense of administering a lethal injection, will probably never be acceptable in Israel, there has been more and more openness to the idea of disconnecting life-support systems. A few years ago, Rabbi Haim David Halevy, late Chief Rabbi of Tel Aviv-Yaffo, agreed to allow disconnecting a ventilator from a terminal patient on the condition that the patient had requested it and was suffering terribly (Halevy 1978). His reasoning was based on the Talmudic idea of "removing the impediment." In Babylonian medicine, it was believed that the exit of the soul from a dying patient could be delayed by placing a grain of salt on the patient's tongue. Although the Talmud did not permit actually killing the patient, it did permit removing the impediment, the grain of salt, in order to allow the patient to die in peace. Halevy reasoned that disconnecting a ventilator was, similarly, only removing an impediment and did not amount to killing. However, when he stated this position at a conference on medical Halacha several years ago, many religious doctors stood on their feet and shouted that he was going against the greatest of authorities. Indeed, his position is only a minority one today. It can be argued whether religious decisions are to proceed like democracy, according to the rule of the majority.

In any case, the Steinberg committee's proposed law on care of the dying patient (Public Committee on the Dying Patient 2002) does not accept Rabbi Halevy's opinion. Instead, they propose to allow refraining from starting ventilation, while forbidding stopping it once it has been started. They do propose allowing ventilation from oxygen bottles, and then deciding not to replace the bottle. They also suggest allowing ventilation controlled by a timer, and then deciding not to reset the timer. Whether these alternatives are really ethically different from disconnecting a ventilator is a question that calls for much philosophical and religious discussion.

Determination of the Moment of Death

Technology that allows terminal patients to be kept for longer and longer periods of time on life-support systems, coupled with advances in major organ transplants, has led in many parts of the world to reconsiderations of the concept of death. Israel is no different in this respect. Although the religious establishment may not always influence many areas of clinical decision making, religious scholars have worked very actively, together with the medical establishment, in developing criteria for determining the moment of death. The Chief Rabbinate accepted the concept of brain stem death quite early. The reasoning is based on the idea that since breathing is the basic condition of life, and since the brain stem controls breathing, brain stem death is biological death (Goren 1992).

The second phrase of the Scripture quoted at the beginning of this chapter refers to our duty to carry out the words of the Torah. However, the meaning of the word of God is sometimes open to debate. There is a very strong segment of religious and nonreligious people in Israel who do not follow the Chief Rabbinate on the matter of brain death, and refuse to accept that someone is dead unless the heart has permanently stopped beating (Steinberg 1994). It seems to be a matter of whether you choose to follow the Bible at Genesis II, 7, which refers to the "breath of life," suggesting that breathing is the defining factor of life, or whether you choose to follow Deuteronomy XII, 23, which says that "the blood is the life," suggesting that one is not dead until the blood stops flowing, i.e., until asystole. In practice, however, rabbinical opinion is quite sophisticated and shows considerable familiarity with medical knowledge.

Truog collected considerable evidence to demonstrate that patients who have been declared brain dead by current clinical criteria have continued brain function of various sorts, including even "hemodynamic response to surgical incisions at the time of organ removal" (Truog and Fackler 1992). In response to critics who claimed that such surviving functions are not "significant," Truog replied: "But if it is a question of significance, why do we place great emphasis on the pupillary light and corneal reflexes (neurologic functions of minimal physiologic significance) and ignore the neurologic regulation of salt and water homeostasis (neurologic functions of critical physiologic significance)?" (Truog 2001: 616).

It seems to have been on the basis of a similar hesitation to declare some brain functions "significant" and others not, that the distinguished and influential Rabbi Shlomo Zalman Auerbach refused to accept that someone is dead until it is proven that every single brain cell is dead (see Steinberg 1994). However, Jewish law forbids disturbing a dying patient. The tests to establish brain death would be highly disturbing if the patient were still alive. The fact that we are carrying out tests, however, shows that we do not yet know whether the patient is alive or dead. The patient might still be alive. Thus, in carrying out the tests, we risk disturbing a dying patient. So Rabbi Auerbach forbade tests for brain death, effectively forbidding taking hearts, lungs, and livers for transplant.

Many secular and religious Israelis alike seem to agree in refusing to accept brain death, as is seen in the low organ donation rates in Israel. Not only do families refuse donation requests, but doctors often fail to comply with a request to donate organs. According to the Israeli Ministry of Health, "Over 1000 people are always waiting for transplants [of various kinds]. The willingness to donate organs in Israel is very low, as compared to the West. The donation response rate in Israel is close to 50 percent, while in other Western countries one finds rates of 60 to 70 percent. In Israel 4 percent of the population hold donor cards as compared to 15 to 35 percent in other Western countries" (Israeli Ministry of Health 2002). This can be too easily attributed to ignorance about brain death, when what we really seem to have is not ignorance but a disagreement about the definitions of life and death. Indeed, it seems unfair to accuse people of ignorance for refusing to accept a modern definition that seems pretty clearly to have been introduced for the specific purpose of making organs available for transplantation.

Israel is similar in this respect to Japan, where heart transplants are also legal, but donations are rare. Japan's 1997 Organ Transplantation Law allows people to choose between brain death and traditional death by writing their preference on a donor card (Morioka 2001). There is a similar law in New Jersey in the United States. Capron objected to such laws on the ground (among others) that they lead "some people to conclude that they should be free to choose between the standards" (Capron 2001: 1244). Such freedom seems ideal for a country like Israel, where we have an old saying that when you have two Jews, you have three opinions. In all seriousness, the liberal principle that we own our own bodies, a principle that is also accepted by some Orthodox rabbis (see Rafael 1992), would suggest that we should be free to decide when, if ever, to donate parts of our bodies. Such a law should also increase the rate of donations. Those who accept brain death would presumably continue to donate no less than before, while those who do not accept it might at least be persuaded to donate more kidneys, corneas, and skin.

There is in Israel some discussion of the idea that people who are not willing to donate their organs and do not carry donor cards should not be allowed to receive organs from others. Given the medical ideal, however, of equal treatment for everyone, it is questionable whether this will ever become law.

It must seem strange to some readers that a situation exists in Israel in which the Chief Rabbinate approves of brain death and major organ transplants, and some rabbis and their followers oppose this policy. Although some people might think of Israel as a religious theocracy, it is a democratic state and Judaism is a democratic religion. There is broad consensus forbidding some practices, such as active euthanasia. On other important issues there is no broad consensus and there are many schools of thought. It should also be pointed out that to permit something is not to say that you have to do it. The Chief Rabbinate, which represents a mainstream majority, gives certificates of *kashrut*, for example, saying in effect that certain foods are permitted. Other persons have stricter standards of slaughter and preparation, and will only eat foods that their own rabbis have approved. Similarly, although the Chief Rabbinate permits the use of accepted standards of brain death, others elect not to take advantage of this permission and to abide by stricter standards, including cardiac death.

Euthanasia, Futile Treatment, Hospices, and Neonatal Intensive Care

Although it is unlikely that active euthanasia will ever be permitted in Israel, one hears anecdotally, especially from nurses, that high doses of morphine are intentionally used as a means of active euthanasia, under the pretense that only the relief of pain was intended. Interviews with experienced physicians, also anecdotal, suggest that the nurses are exaggerating or misinterpreting what they see. The word "anecdotal" has been used repeatedly here, in order to draw attention to the fact that no serious research seems as yet to have been done on this subject. In fact, it is hard to imagine that any hospital would allow such research to be conducted within its walls.

Although discontinuation of futile treatment is sometimes called passive euthanasia, the association with any form of killing is unfair and misleading. Discontinuing futile treatment is an inseparable part of medicine in Israel as elsewhere. This is most obvious in hospices, where aggressive treatment of the fatal disease is stopped, but other diseases are treated and everything possible is done to relieve pain and increase comfort. In Israel we have both hospice institutions and a home hospice system in which the family cares for the patient with nursing and medical support.

A well-known Israeli hospice is the Saint Louis Hospital (popularly known as the "French Hospital") in Jerusalem, which is run by Roman Catholic nuns and volunteers and recognized by the Israeli Ministry of Health. Although run by Catholics, it serves kosher food because of the many Orthodox Jewish patients. The devotion and kindness of the sisters and volunteers have done much toward changing the attitudes of Orthodox Jews, who have traditionally distrusted Christians because of the Crusades, the Inquisition, and persecutions in Europe. Their view of their patients is illustrated by the following incident. In an interview with the manageress, Sister Lucy, some years ago, we used the phrase "terminal patient." Sister Lucy replied: "If you use that phrase again, the interview will be over. How do you know that you are less terminal than they are? You can walk out of here and get hit by a car, while they can continue to live for a long time. We have even sent people home from here."

Discontinuing futile treatment is also an inseparable part of neonate intensive care, a specialty that is highly developed in Israel. This specialty cannot advance unless efforts are made to save more and more difficult cases. However, this naturally leads to numbers of cases in which well-intentioned efforts turn out to have been futile and a decision may have to be made to stop treatment. In these decisions, nurses may have an especially important role. Neonate intensive care unit (ICU) treatment requires constant nursing supervision and care of the baby; therefore the nurse naturally knows the patient much more intimately than the doctors do. The nurse's opinion is therefore listened to. When the doctor is not willing to listen, the nurse can call in the chief ward sister for support. One distinguished Israeli neonatologist has predicted that the nurses will eventually run the neonate ICUs, and the doctors will only be consultants.

As in the neonate ICU, so in adult medicine, the patient's primary contact with health care is the nurse. Although bioethical discussions of end-of-life care may emphasize dramatic acts like injecting high doses of morphine, or disconnecting ventilators, end-of-life care of real patients in real hospitals is more a matter of routine nursing procedures, such as moving the patient regularly to avoid bedsores, bathing, changing clothing, and sanitation. Here, as in other aspects of end-of-life care, there are no laws, few guidelines, and little consensus. When it becomes a question of moving the patient to avoid bedsores or refraining from doing so because this might disturb and endanger the patient, the nurse often must rely on her or his individual judgment and conscience.

As on other matters discussed in this chapter, the authors are divided on whether the need for and practice of individual judgment is a healthy situation. Leavitt, a philosopher and bioethicist, believes pluralism to be the only reasonable approach in a situation where there are so many unknowns, and sees Israeli lack of order as making this pluralism possible. In contrast, Amidror, a clinical nurse, believes that clinical staff and physicians, as well as nurses, are in need of more order and clearer guidelines.

References

Capron, A. M. 2001. "Brain Death—Well Settled Yet Still Unresolved" (editorial). *New England Journal of Medicine* 344: 1244–1246.

Eidelman, L. A., D. J. Jacobson, R. Pizov, D. Gerber, L. Leibovitz, and C. L. Sprung. 1998. "Foregoing Life-sustaining Treatment in an Israeli ICU." *Intensive Care Medicine* 24: 162–166.

Goren, S. 1991. "The Use of Medicines and Doctors: A Commandment or a Right?" *Harefua* 121: 58–60 (Hebrew).

Goren, S. 1992. "Brain Death Is the End of Life According to Halacha." *Hatzofey*, August 21, p. 5 (in Hebrew).

Halevy, H. D. 1978. Aseh Lecha Rav (Halachic questions and answers). *Tel Aviv*, II, 39–40 (in Hebrew).

Israeli Ministry of Health, National Center for Transplantation. 2002. http://www.health.gov.il/transplant/trumat_nechunut.htm (accessed April 15, 2004) (in Hebrew).

Morioka, M. 2001. "Reconsidering Brain Death: A Lesson from Japan's Fifteen Years of Experience." *Hastings Center Report* 31: 41–46.

Public Committee on the Dying Patient. 2002. Proposed Law on the Dying Patient (in Hebrew).

Rafael, S. 1992. *Coercive Medical Treatment. Proceedings of the 33rd Conference on the Oral Tora (Tora Sh'baal Pe)*. Jerusalem: Mossad HaRav Kook, pp. 74–81 (in Hebrew).

Shalev, C., and G. Hildesheimer. 2001. *Medical Treatment at the End of Life: Proposals for a Normative Standard*. Tel Hashomer: The Gertner Institute (in Hebrew).

Steinberg, A. 1994. "Determination of the Moment of Death: Survey of Positions." *Assia* 14: 5–16 (in Hebrew).

Truog, R. D., 2001. "The Diagnosis of Brain Death" (correspondence). *New England Journal of Medicine* 345: 616–618.

Truog, R. D., and J. C. Fackler. 1992. "Rethinking Brain Death." *Critical Care Medicine* 20: 1705–1712.

Wenger, N. S., O. Golan, C. Shalev, and S. Glick. 2002. " Hospital Ethics Committees in Israel: Structure, Function and Heterogeneity in the Setting of Statutory Ethics Committees." *Journal of Medical Ethics* 28: 177–182.

7

End-of-Life Care in Japan

Darryl Macer

Japan has a history that goes back at least three millennia and a culture that shows great respect for aged persons, so one could expect it to treat the elderly well when they are dying. The problem in Japan for end-of-life care is not so much a lack of resources or attention, but too much attention to the goals of sustaining life, without enough attention being given to the wishes of the patient as a person.

Japan has developed some of its own medical ethics, merging Buddhist and Confucian rules into a Shinto background with a recent importation of Western values (Macer 1999; 2003). Japanese ethics could be said to be now rather pragmatic and centered on the authorities. There is universal health insurance, which supports the concept of social justice and access for all to health care supported by taxes. Although the principle of justice is accepted socially, the increasing proportion of aged persons means sick people are expected to pay a slightly higher proportion of the medical costs themselves to lessen the tax burden. While the sick expect to be covered by this insurance, most do not want to be a burden on the state or family. Informed consent is becoming accepted, and bioethics is part of a transition that is transforming Japanese society from a paternalistic to an individualistic one.

Cultural Factors

Since the fifth and sixth centuries A.D., the medical profession in Japan has been restricted to the privileged classes. With the centralization of government in the seventh and eighth centuries, a bureau of medicine was established, with the Yoro penal and civil codes creating an official physician class. After the Heian period (800–1200 A.D.), the government-sponsored health service was replaced by professional physicians.

In the sixteenth century, a code of practice called the "Seventeen Rules of Enjuin" was drawn up that is very similar to the Hippocratic code. This code, developed by practitioners of the Ri-shu school, also emphasized a priestly role for the physician. The physicians "should always be kind to people.... [they] should always be devoted to loving people." There is a very strong paternalistic attitude by doctors even today (Hamano 2003). The code also has a directive to keep the art secret and to be concerned about quacks. No abortives are allowed, or poisons. The code contains a number of rules for virtue, such as, "You should rescue even such patients as you dislike or hate" and "You should be delighted if, after treating a patient without success, the patient receives medicine from another physician, and is cured."

Since the Meiji restoration in the nineteenth century, the doors of Japan have been opened to all countries. Recently, traditional ideas have undergone rapid change with globalization, itself driven by the communications devices that Japanese industry has exported around the world. Modern Western medicine took hold in Asia in the nineteenth century. The rapid progress of medical technology has led to challenges in the way that medicine is practiced. The existing systems and patterns that are seen in the relationships among patients, families, health professionals, and the society in general are being changed. At the same time, as the technology is transferred, some values are also imported. These are not just the modern global cultural view that new technology must be better than old.

The black episode in Japanese medical ethics is the experiments conducted on prisoners in Manchuria, while China was under Japanese occupation in World War II. At least 3,000 persons, mainly Chinese, were murdered by or after vivisection and other experiments in facilities under Japanese Imperial Army Unit 731 at several locations in China. The activities included vivisection practice for newly qualified army surgeons, intentional infection, trials of nonstandardized treatments, and tests to discover the tolerances of the human body (Tsuchiya 2000). In contrast to the German preoccupation with their war crimes, neither Japanese nor

Chinese bioethics has sufficiently analyzed these experiments and the ethical issues they raise (Morioka 2000; Tsuchiya 2000; Macer 2001; Nie 2001). Because of the opportunity to have access to the best medical research facilities in Asia, many physicians went to the unit. It was not until the mid-1990s that some members of the unit started to confess and apologize for their actions as they reached old age. However, the discussion of the issues in bioethics has only just begun. Since the best medical students often trained in unit 731 because it was the best-equipped research laboratory in Asia at the time, the preoccupation with technical as opposed to moral and spiritual issues of medicine is consistent with the mentality of medical experimentation that lead to such extremes.

Currently, Japanese medical ethics is changing, and a diversity of views similar to those in Western medical ethics are being debated. The hesitant introduction of patient-centered decision making is related more to the structure of Japanese society than to any difference in an individual's attitudes between Japanese and Western societies. This can be shown from the results of opinion surveys. For example, when individuals were asked to give the reasons for their opinions on bioethical issues such as genetic manipulation or screening, there was at least as much variety in opinions expressed by members of the general public in Japan as there is in other countries (Macer 1994a).

Since the 1970s, people have become more conscious of their right to informed consent, which could be attributed to the importation of civil rights debates that occurred in the United States and Japan in the 1960s (Kimura 1995). The concept of human rights was recognized in the constitutions of the Meiji era in the nineteenth century and that following World War II. Article 13 of the Japanese constitution guarantees each adult individual's right to self-determination. This has been interpreted by the courts to include the right to refuse life-sustaining care and medical intervention, including refusal of blood transfusion by adults. However, in general practice this is often ignored, and only in the past few years have courts applied that concept to patient's decision making. In the nineteenth century, some philosophers, such as Nakae Chomin, introduced concepts of human rights (Hamano 1997). He reinterpreted Confucianism by injecting concepts of popular sovereignty and democratic equality, and provided an internal tradition of human rights. I

(Macer 1999) would place the origin of informed choice with the older samurai tradition, which includes the control of when one will die and the dignity of honorable suicide choices. In addition, the concept of informed consent is seen in the writings of Hanaoka Seishu on breast cancer from the nineteenth century.

With the introduction of Western medicine, there has also been an influx of Western religion, philosophy, and etiquette. As cultures evolve, it becomes impossible to separate which aspects were introduced from which sources at which time. Within a few decades, a culture may see something as unique to its own tradition even though it was imported. Even the concept of having a written text can be a cultural import in some Asian countries. Although ancient Japanese and Chinese books date back more than 1300 years, and legal systems were established at earlier times, the Westernization of Asia led to European-style laws being introduced. This affects the types of laws and guidelines that govern medical practice. The concept of natural death is mixed in Japan (Lock 1995).

The term "bioethics" has had the effect of stimulating cultures around the world to think about the relationships between patient and practitioner, as well as between the public and the government (Macer 1994b). One reaction to the introduction of Western medical ethics, particularly from the United States in the 1980s, has been a backlash claiming that Japanese are different from Westerners. This argument can be used to defend existing practices or to slow down rapid social change. The development of the Asian Bioethics Association is one attempt to break with the domination of U.S. bioethics. At the United Nations Educational, Scientific and Cultural Organization's 1997 Asian Bioethics Conference (Fujiki and Macer 1998), there was discussion by a number of Asian researchers on the need to recognize traditional Asian bioethics rather than importing bioethics from the United States. There has been discussion on whether the idea of fundamental human rights is compatible with the Asian ethos (Sakamoto 1999).

Important Medical Institutions

Currently, professional responsibility is outlined by laws and guidelines. In Japan, there are several basic laws, including the Doctor's Act. The

Japan Medical Association (JMA) approved the concept of informed consent in 1991, which superseded the Physician's Code of Ethics of 1951, which was more paternalistic (Kimura 1995). There are professional guidelines issued for members of academic societies to follow, but they can still practice medicine outside of the professional society. Consensus is often more important than passing a law (Bai et al. 1987; Shinagawa 2000).

Physicians are required to obtain consent to medical treatment according to the 1971 Medical Practitioner's Act, Article 23. The obligation for treatment is based on assessing what can reasonably be expected in view of the knowledge and experience that characterizes the average physician. The obligation for consent means that the patient's will is to be respected when medical opinions are divided as to the necessity of the treatment. Arbitrary administration of medical care violates Articles 204 and 205 of the criminal code. Article 202 of the criminal code forbids a person to help in another person's suicide.

The Council of Medical Ethics, established under the provisions of Article 25 of the Medical Practitioner's Act, is an advisory body supervised by the Minister of Public Welfare and consists of the presidents of the Japan Medical Association, the Japanese Dental Association, and scholars and staffs from related administrative departments. It functions to take administrative measures to eliminate physicians and dentists who commit malpractice or act unethically. Article 211 of the penal code states that if a physician injures a patient and the injuries cause death by mistreatment, the physician is liable for up to 5 years' imprisonment and/ or up to a 500,000-yen fine (US$4500). According to Article 7–2 of the Physicians Law, if a doctor is sentenced to imprisonment or a fine, the Ministry of Health, Labor and Welfare (MHLW) can remove his license or suspend his practice for a certain period of time. This action follows the decision of the Medical Practice Council according to Article 7–4. However, in practice, many Japanese are still reluctant to seek damages for malpractice (Feldman 1985; Bai 1983).

There are separate laws outlining the activities of health professionals, including physicians, dentists, nurses, acupuncturists, masseurs, and other health care professionals. Nonregistered professionals are not allowed to work. In 1990, there were 210,197 registered physicians working in Japan, a ratio of 170 per 100,000 population. The Medical Practitioner's

Act of 1971 contains guidelines on what physicians should and should not do. There are some common exceptions to the law in practice. For example, Article 17 of the act forbids nonregistered persons from performing an action that might present harm to another person's body if not done by a sufficiently sound medical technique. This would outlaw taking blood pressure or performing ear piecing. However, these actions are commonly performed everywhere. This law could be applied to those who hastened the death of a person by an apparatus. The curriculum for medical training is set by the Ministry of Education, but physicians are licensed after passing a national exam by the MHLW.

The Medical Service Law and the Health Center Law are two important laws in a series that control the operation of medical facilities. In 1991, there were 10,066 hospitals in Japan. About 81 percent of Japan's hospitals are privately operated. They tend to be smaller than the public sector hospitals, and many are developed from physician-owned family practices. A physician's referral is not required for admission to a hospital.

In 1991, there were 82,118 general clinics in Japan. Clinics are the usual name for physicians' offices and about 94 percent are privately operated. A clinic cannot keep a patient for more than 48 hours and is legally defined as having fewer than 20 beds, whereas a hospital has 20 or more beds. About 60 percent of clinics have no accommodation for patients, but they are usually well equipped. Physicians in clinics do not have access to hospital facilities and must refer patients to hospitals if they cannot provide the services on site. The clinics compete with hospitals for the patients, who can choose what they prefer.

There are very few social workers in Japan, with an average of 0.2 per 100 beds in general hospitals and 0.5 per 100 beds in mental hospitals in 1991. However, there are efforts under way to increase this. Insurance programs do not recognize counseling and psychotherapy as methods of medical treatment to be reimbursed. This means that counselors are encouraged to see as many people as possible a day and have many short visits, which also is a general problem of dental and medical care in Japan.

In 1998, the government altered the law to allow physicians some compensation for taking the extra time that is needed to seek informed consent (Macer, 2003). The obligation for consent means that the patient's will is to be respected when medical opinions are divided as to the necessity of the treatment (Tokyo District Court 1971). The patient must be competent; a person over 15 years is considered competent in most cases. For infants and the mentally ill, the consent of the person exercising parental authority is required. A Tokyo District Court in 1992 upheld a case brought against Tokyo University Medical School involving informed consent. The operation was a medical success, but the patient was not informed of the chances of failure and brought a case against the hospital. However, in other cases since then, the courts did not uphold informed consent (Swinbanks 1989; Tanida 1991). In practice, the concept of fully informed consent is still being introduced into Japanese medical practice.

Consent and Decision Making

Who Decides?

While the consent concept is well established, there are important questions about who gives consent. The evolution of the concept of patient autonomy is seen in a trend that is reflected in all Asian cultures moving from paternalistic compassion and love toward informed decision making. The situation is more difficult than simply claiming that in the past patients did not have autonomy and that physicians always acted paternalistically. The sick may prefer to leave the decisions up to others or use subtle linguistic expressions to convey their will. However, there is still a hierarchical social system that makes it difficult for patient and doctor to be truly at an equal level in their relationship. Even more so, the concept of informed choice, where the patient becomes the consumer of medicine, is seen in the pharmacy stores but not in the medical consultation. Many sick persons are afraid to be a bother or burden to others, so they attempt to avoid trouble that could occur if they clearly expressed their will and it differed from that of others.

There are also theories of ethics in the West as well as the East based on community, which argue that individuality, autonomy, or the rights of a person are not suited to the community structure of society. Communitarians argue that societies need a commitment to general welfare and common purpose, and this protects their members against the abuses of individualism, which could be equated with a selfish pursuit of liberty.

Regarding the principles of bioethics in Japan, harmony has been discussed as a potential overriding principle, but it is unclear if there really is any one principle that dominates (Macer 1994a; 1998). Some commentators believe that autonomy is not seen in Japan, but the moral principle of autonomy is applied to many people in decision-making regarding life choices that are bioethical dilemmas.

Right to Privacy

While privacy is regarded as a high virtue in some countries in law, like Japan, there are common exceptions in practice. For example, while the Tokyo government issued guidance that employer tests for HIV can only be conducted with the informed consent of the employees, the Tokyo police department was found guilty in court of secretly testing potential recruits for HIV.

The involvement of the family in medical decision making means that some modern Western ideas on confidentiality are not yet accepted in Asian medical practice. The family may be told medical news earlier than the patient. In Japan, many sick persons who know they have a terminal illness play a "game of avoiding to hurting another," pretending they do not know the seriousness of the disease with family members, who in turn pretend the patient is not terminally ill. Modern Asian society, however, is individualistic in many aspects, and patients' rights are being promoted by many persons. Japanese medical ethics is in a transitional phase that cannot be separated from broader socioeconomic changes. The late twentieth century has seen rapid change in the concepts of how a person is integrated into the family and the boundaries of the family with whom one dwells (Maekawa and Macer 1999).

Privacy of communication is guaranteed in the constitution. Article 21 guarantees freedom of assembly and association as well as freedom of speech, press, and all other forms of expression. There is the Law on the Protection of Computer Information on Individuals, which applies to the handling of information on individuals that is processed and stored in computers by government agencies. The law states that government agencies are prohibited from using the information for purposes other than the original purpose for which the files were compiled. Any person may require a government agency to disclose his or her information stored in the computer, and, if necessary, demand its alteration. This could be interpreted to mean that the truth of any health information entered into a computer must be revealed following a request by the person to whom it applies. If someone gives others an individual's medical data (for example, giving the result of a genetic screening test to an employer), Section 134–1 of the penal code could apply. If the person who leaked the information is a national employee, the Law on Government Employees could punish them. The Occupational Health and Safety Law obligates the health care staff to keep secrets. Moreover, under Articles 14 and 15 of the AIDS law, the person who leaks this secret will be punished beyond the penal code. Article 15 sets penalties of up to 6 months' imprisonment or up to a 200,000-yen fine (US$1900).

Asai (2002) illustrated the problems encountered in the clinical setting when treating a senile demented patient in Japan. He argued that although existing ethical guidelines and procedures are ordinarily quite useful, ethical decisions based on them could sometimes be inconclusive because uncertainty inherent to real-life situations such as the care of a demented elderly patient exist. His conclusion was an ethical approach to keep listening to others, keep thinking what is good with humility, and keep questioning the ethical validity of what we have done and what we will do in the name of the patient's benefit.

Advance Directives

The Japan Society for Death with Dignity was established in 1976, and after failing to introduce a law on the withdrawal of life-sustaining therapy, it promoted the use of living wills. Living wills are not common, and less than 1 percent of persons die with some form of advance directive. There is no case of a doctor being sued in the courts for following a living will, but there are examples where doctors and families together may disagree with the living will. Members of the society seldom report a case where a physician does not respect a living will (Akabayashi 2002).

Public opinion surveys find strong public support for the concept of death with dignity. Although in a 1995 survey 80 percent of the persons said they were aware of living wills, 88 percent said that they would give a lot of leeway to surrogates to override the decision (Akabayashi et al. 1999). The main reasons given were that it was difficult to talk about death and dying in the family, trust in their families, and that it was difficult to imagine the future. However, research indicates that people in East Asian cultures do not want to talk freely about death inside the family, and few have considered preparing advance directives (Hsin and Macer 2003).

Physicians, however, are more supportive of attempting life-sustaining treatment (Asai et al. 1995). The surveys show that people do want to die with dignity, but that there are difficulties in expressing these views to those around them. More important, physicians usually lack the communication skills to talk about the options with patients, so that they may decide to start and continue life-sustaining treatment rather than question whether the patients want it. The views of university physicians caring for adult patients at an academic medical center concerning advance directives were surveyed in 1996. Almost all respondents chose the option of having the doctor and family decide on the treatment for demented patients (Macer et al. 1996; Rothenberg et al. 1996). The persons chosen to discuss the treatment with consisted of a mixture of relatives and those caring for the patient, and those in the family who had the best ability to decide. The respondents said that the most important factor in making the decision was what is considered best for the patient, followed by the family's will.

In a survey of the ethics committees at university hospitals (all 80 have ethics committees) in 1996, it was found that only 4 percent had discussed cessation of treatment and only 6 percent had discussed euthanasia or death with dignity (Fukatsu et al. 1997), which means that ethics committees seldom discuss these issues. A more recent survey also found that few bioethics discussions occur in ethics committees (Shirai 2003). The physician, nurse, and family are the main persons who discuss the end-of-life care, if anyone does. Do-not-resuscitate orders are not common (Fukaura et al. 1995).

Age is one factor in the acceptance of withdrawal of aggressive treatment in discussions that patients will have in their family. However, many hospitals may seek to reap profits by having old persons in their intensive care units, even after death. Not accepting brain death as a criterion means that extra days or weeks of intensive care payments can be received by the hospital. There are little data on this practice because most hospitals do not like to publicize such a disrespectful act. Doing so would upset the families and lead to a loss of revenue. However, there is still a tendency to be less aggressive in treatment the older the person is, which is consistent with older traditions that aged persons should not be a burden on the family when their time is up.

Context of End-of-Life Care

A majority of persons in Japan die in a hospital unless it is a sudden death, in part because there are relatively few nursing homes in Japan compared with Western countries. One of the reasons for the relatively low number is that bedridden elderly persons over 65 years of age can receive low-cost medical treatment, including hospitalization, and anyone over 70 years of age is eligible for free care. Government-supported Health Services Facilities for the Elderly were established by The Amendment of the Act for Health and Medical Service for the Elderly. The facilities must be staffed with medical doctors, nurses, nursing care staff, physiotherapists or occupational therapists, health consultants, and nutritionists. The municipalities pay the medical expenses, while the elderly bear the cost of personal items such as meals, diapers, haircuts, and daily necessities.

The first palliative care unit opened in 1981 and by 2001 there were 79 such units or hospices in Japan. Although at the beginning these units were Buddhist or Christian, the majority are now nonreligious. Only 2 percent of cancer patients die in such units (Akabayashi 2002), which means only 1 percent of total deaths. The low use of these may be related to the lack of facilities and also to some social reluctance for the families to use them. About half the cancer patients may not be told that they even have cancer (Elwyn et al. 2002), although many guess their disease, especially when it is at an advanced stage.

The Ministry of Health, Labor and Welfare and the Japan Medical Association have published manuals to help practitioners resolve other difficult dilemmas (Japan Medical Association 1989; Akabayashi et al. 1999). The manual on euthanasia includes chapters on two central issues, truth telling and pain control. In the preface, the manual states:

Mere life prolonging treatment for terminally ill patients should be reconsidered in terms of respect for human dignity as well as the psychological burden for the family in question. For example, cardiopulmonary resuscitation for cardiac arrest or respiratory cessation of terminal patients often results in mere lengthening of the patient's suffering.... From now on, patients' will and rights of self-determination should be respected in this area of medical care. (translation from Akabayashi 2002: 520)

The JMA manual on cancer lists four factors that should be taken into account when considering whether to disclose a diagnosis of cancer: (1) the purpose of disclosure should be clear; (2) the patient and family members need to be able to accept the diagnosis; (3) the nature of the relationship between the practitioner and the family and patient should be considered; and (4) psychological support should be provided to the patient after disclosure. However, there is general reluctance to tell the truth about terminal illness in Japan, although the trend is for a growing percentage of doctors to say that they do so and for a growing percentage of the public to say that they want to know. Even in 1980, 61 percent of people said that they would like to be told the truth, and in 1981 only 27 percent of doctors said that they would never tell patients the truth. In 1989 a government task force concluded that the truth should be told, and that view is, in principle, official.

Pain management is inadequate in Japan, but the situation is improving. Japanese physicians have been reluctant to administer morphine because of tough laws on related drugs. The Narcotics and Psychotropics Law was amended in 1990 to improve the accessibility of morphine preparations to cancer patients with pain. The MHLW edited four volumes for palliative care with guidelines on cancer pain relief and legislative management of narcotics use in hospital, clinics, and pharmacies (Takeda 1991). Morphine use in pain management increased 17-fold between 1979 and 1989 owing to attitude changes in physicians regarding pain management. This use increased further after the law was changed in 1990 and more physicians accepted the need to alleviate pain in terminal care. Morphine has been changed from an illegal drug to an accepted pain treatment, following the World Health Organization's Cancer Relief Program in 1980. In 1989 the MHLW legalized the use of 10-mg tablets of slow-release morphine (MS Contin) and 30-mg tablets in 1990. The amount of morphine consumed is still only one-fourth of

U.S. levels and one-eighth of U.K. levels, which is in contrast to the reverse relationships for most other pharmaceutical products.

Public surveys in the 1990s found that 80 percent of those surveyed do not want treatment continued if they are in a vegetative state, and 75 percent said that they do not want treatment if in pain and close to death. People over 70 years of age were more willing to have treatment continued. However, the euthanasia cases expose the inadequacies of Japanese terminal care, where many patients who have pain remain in pain because pain-killing drugs are not fully covered by the national health insurance. This creates the desire to die, and when combined with inadequate medical communication and trust between patient and doctor, there will remain relatively high (about 50 percent) public support for informed and consenting active euthanasia of competent patients, despite its illegality.

The Japanese Geriatric Society for the Terminal Care in the Elderly issued a position paper on terminal care for the elderly (Uemura et al. 2000). In particular, it prohibited discrimination merely on the grounds of old age. Examples of the statements include the following:

Position statement No. 1: Ageism should be rejected. Appropriate health care should be guaranteed for severely demented persons as an inviolable fundamental human right.

Position statement No. 2: The values and preferences of the elderly patients should guide the terminal care that the patients have unless their values and wishes are inconsistent with social morality.

Position statement No. 3: Terminal care should be regarded as one subspecialty made up mainly of palliative care medicine. It should be aimed at improving the quality of life of the patients.

Position statement No. 4: Terminal care for the elderly should include the care for the patient's family. When the patients lose the capacity for self-determination, the patient's family plays an important role in decision-making. (translation from Asai 2000: 136)

Issues in Euthanasia and Physician-Assisted Suicide

In the absence of a specific law regarding end-of-life care or bioethics, case law becomes more important in Japan (Macer 2003). There have been several cases dealing with active euthanasia by family members and by doctors since a 1949 case in the Tokyo District Court. The first six cases involved euthanasia by family members, and in each case they were found guilty of "homicide upon request" and received suspended sentences (Akabayashi 2002). The judges' statements provide some guidance, but are not the same as Japanese law. They do, however, establish legal precedent. A medical treatment to reduce or remove pain that may also cause a premature death is considered lawful under several conditions:

1. The patient suffers from an incurable disease as judged from contemporary medical knowledge and technology, and death is impending;

2. Physical pain is unbearably extreme and without any other means of relief;

3. There is consent or a contract based on the true will of the suffering person. In the case where the consciousness of the patient is not clear enough to express his wishes and there is no hope of recovery, the consent or earnest request of the immediate family is sufficient; and

4. A generally practiced medical act is to be employed to this end. (Nagoya High Court 1962, 12.22)

The Japan Medical Association recommended that there be general legislation allowing doctors to withdraw life-sustaining treatment if patients wish it to be done in cases of terminal illness. The JMA wants the law to recognize living wills, but they oppose legalizing euthanasia. The report by the JMA bioethics committee also suggested that cancer patients be informed of their disease "in principle."

A Japanese court also decided that a man who helped his terminally ill female partner die in response to her requests in 1991 did so out of deep love, and he was only sentenced to 1 year in prison, with a 2-year stay of execution. There is greater punishment for physicians who assist death. In a 1991 case of physician-assisted active euthanasia in Japan, a doctor at Tokai University injected potassium chloride into an incompetent patient at the pleading of relatives. The university's ethics committee judged it unethical. There are mixed opinions among physicians on the issue (Macer et al. 1996). In 1995 there was a ruling by the Yokohama District Court on the Tokai University case, which described four legal requirements for physician-assisted voluntary euthanasia:

1. The patient must be suffering from unbearable physical pain.

2. The patient's death must be unavoidable and imminent.

3. Every possible palliative treatment and care to ease the patient's physical pain and suffering must have been provided, and no alternatives must be available.

4. The patient must have expressed a clear and voluntary desire to have his or her life shortened.

In the 1995 case only the second requirement was considered to have been met; thus the physician was found guilty of homicide and sentenced to 2 years' imprisonment (Macer 1996; Hamano 2003).

Handicapped neonates are usually treated aggressively, with the physicians making decisions. The general view is that the parents are distraught and unable to decide. Even hopeless cases may be more aggressively treated than in most Western countries. This is in contrast to the traditional custom of *mabiki,* which was to leave handicapped newborns to die. There have been no legal suits regarding the withdrawal of treatment for handicapped neonates. A survey of consultant pediatricians found that 90 percent would intensively treat a Down syndrome baby, even if the parents refused treatment, but 90 percent of the public would not consider a doctor who failed to treat a handicapped infant as a murderer. Similarly, often there is hesitation to discontinue treatment of demented patients (Asai and Ohnishi 2001).

The surveys of nurses and physicians that have been conducted in Japan provide a range of results, but in the widest survey, half of the nurses and doctors responded that they have been asked at some point for voluntary euthanasia (Asai et al. 2001). In that 1999 survey, 88 percent of doctors and 85 percent of nurses answered that the request can sometimes be rational, but only 33 percent of doctors and 23 percent of nurses responded that it was ethically right, and 23 percent of doctors and 22 percent of nurses said that they would help the patient commit euthanasia. Only the doctors, however, admitted having performed voluntary euthanasia.

Organ Transplants from Brain-Dead Donors

One of the most controversial technologies in Asian countries is organ transplantation. In some ways, organ transplantation was a symbolic issue for the introduction of a bioethics debate into Japan (Macer 1992), and thus this specific technology may have led to consideration of the need for the public to be involved in the debate on medical ethics. The issue of consent was closely linked to this question, and it again raised questions of whether people can trust doctors. Rather than religious views, the fundamental doubt in people's minds may have been, and may still be, trust in the medical profession (Macer 1992).

The most controversial issue involving the use of modern scientific technology in Japan is organ transplantation from brain-dead donors. On this issue, there has been more debate in Japan than in any other country in the world. The first heart transplant was performed in 1968; the second was delayed by this debate until 1998 (Morioka 2001; Lock 2002; Bagheri 2003). The brain-death law was passed in 1997, and by mid-2003 there had been 35 transplants approved under the new law. For a country of 125 million people, that is almost insignificant. There are still critics of the law permitting organ transplants from brain-dead donors (Becker 1999). One of the arguments used to support organ donation is love of others. The organ donor cards in Japan feature four little angels (actually a Western concept) giving organs to save others.

A law enabling cornea transplantation was passed in 1958. This law, which allows physicians in general to transplant corneas from cadavers, requires the prior written consent of the family of the dead donor, but does not require consent when there is no surviving family. In 1979, the Act Concerning the Transplantation of Cornea and Kidneys was passed. The level of kidney donation (at least the reported level) has dropped in the past few years with the high profile of the brain-death issue and fear of litigation. A survey of Japan's women's hospitals reported that from 1980 to 1985, 96 of 314 kidneys were obtained from brain-dead donors, and in 1984 to 1988, 152 of 429 kidneys were from brain-dead donors.

The prime minister's ad hoc Committee on Brain Death and Organ Transplantation report of January 1992 unanimously recommended that organ transplants from brain-dead donors who have positively expressed a desire to donate organs should be permitted. It also said that no organ transplants should be performed for patients who have said they do not want to give organs. The committee concluded that organs can be donated if family members agree that the deceased expressed a wish to donate organs and that there has been no pressure on the relatives to make this decision. They recommended that a third party (unnamed) should look at these cases to ensure there is no undue pressure to consent. In addition to these unanimous findings, a majority agreed that brain death is biological human death. A minority of four members said that brain death is close to human death.

Actually, since the mid-1980s, the level of public agreement has been similar to the range of general opinion in Western countries, with about 25 percent rejecting organ transplants from brain-dead donors. It was argued that the Japanese have special cultural barriers to such donations (Lock 2002), an argument that has been questioned by Japanese sociologists and religious groups (Nudeshima 1991). In every culture, some people reject the removal of organs from bodies, and their views should be respected. As mentioned, the more serious doubt in the minds of some people is whether they can trust doctors (Macer 1992), and among ten countries in the Asia-Pacific area surveyed in 1993, Japan had the lowest trust in doctors (Macer 1994a).

The Future of Japanese Bioethics

The key turning point issue for bioethics in Japan was the unprecedented social debate over the law to allow organ transplants from brain-dead donors. It is rare to see a debate between the public and the policy makers over any issue, but this issue led to the introduction of informed consent and the need for medical policy to be more sensitive to public concerns. Patients' rights have been increasing (Macer 1992; Annas and Miller 1994; Morikawa 1994). Japan is in the midst of a transition from paternalism to informed consent to informed choice (Macer 1994b). In fact, the example of the samurai tradition in Japan, which was an informed-choice society, could be used to stimulate future developments for patient empowerment.

The Japanese health care system provides an equitable level of health care coverage using a low proportion of the gross domestic product. In a national survey in 1985 asking persons who had experienced an illness why they had not seen a physician, only 0.4 percent gave economic reasons. This suggests that almost no one is prevented from seeking medical care for economic reasons. There is a complex mesh of insurance systems to cover all persons; the major critic of this arrangement has been the JMA, which has suggested one universal system. Other critics suggest that a universal system might be too rigid to allow proper competition. The current system is based on the ethical presumption of universal coverage for equivalent services, which is being challenged by the aging population and the gradual introduction of more "user" fees (Watts 2000). Nevertheless, the principle of universal coverage is unlikely to be challenged in the foreseeable future.

The bioethics debate may be the catalyst required to transform Japan from a "paternalistic democracy" into one in which the individual has a greater voice in health care decisions. People of any country may resist the rapid change and globalization of their ethics, ideals, and paradigms because ethnic and national identities may be changed or lost, especially in countries with a long history of culture. How countries should approach globalization is a fundamental question, but many individuals in countries with access to common news media have already answered the question by their life-styles and values. To the extent that human rights and the environment are more respected, this trend is to be encouraged.

When Japan opened its doors to Western society in the nineteenth century, it led to the introduction of a newly emerging science and scientific paradigm, but only part of the fabric of Western society. Meanwhile, Western society has continued to evolve, and bioethics has emerged as a result. It is now time for bioethics to be developed in Japan. Part of this development includes importing and developing ethical approaches that can be debated, but a more important part is involving the public in discussion and development of a bioethics policy that takes into account the country's diverse ethical traditions.

References

Akabayashi, A., M. D. Fetters, and T. S. Elwyn. 1999. "Family Consent, Communication, and Advance Directives for Cancer Disclosure: A Japanese Case and Discussion." *Journal of Medical Ethics* 25 (4): 296–301.

Akabayashi, A. 2002. "Euthanasia, Assisted Suicide, and Cessation of Life Support: Japan's Policy, Law, and an Analysis of Whistle Blowing in Two Recent Mercy Killing Cases." *Social Science and Medicine* 55: 517–527.

Annas, G. J., and F. H. Miller. 1994. "The Empire of Death: How Culture and Economics Affect Informed Consent in the U.S., the UK and Japan." *American Journal of Law and Medicine* 20: 357–394.

Asai, A. 2002. "Unknowability and Humility in Clinical Ethical Decisions." *Eubios Journal of Asian and International Bioethics* 12: 133–137.

Asai, A., and M. Ohnishi. 2001. "Reasons for Discontinuation of Treatments for Severely Demented Patients: A Japanese Physician's View." *Eubios Journal of Asian and International Bioethics* 11: 141–144.

Asai, A., S. Fukuhara, and B. Lo. 1995. "Attitudes of Japanese and Japanese-American Physicians Towards Life-sustaining Treatment." *Lancet* 346: 356–359.

Asai, A., M. Ohnishi, S. K. Nagata, N. Tanida, and Y. Yamazaki. 2001. "Doctors' and Nurses' Attitudes Towards and Experiences of Voluntary Euthanasia: Survey of Members of the Japanese Association of Palliative Medicine." *Journal of Medical Ethics* 27: 324–330.

Bagheri, A. 2003. "Criticism of 'Brain Death' Policy in Japan. *Kennedy Institute of Ethics Journal* 13 (4): 359–372.

Bai, K. ed. 1983. *Iryo to Hou to Rinri* (Medicine, Law and Ethics). Tokyo: Iwanamishoten.

Bai, K., Y. Shirai, and M. Ishii. 1987. "In Japan, Consensus Has Limits," *Hastings Center Report* (June) (special suppl.), 18–20.

Becker, C. 1999. "Money Talks, Money Kills—The Economics of Transplantation in Japan and China." *Bioethics* 13 (3): 236–243.

Elwyn, T. D., M. D. Fetters, H. Sasaki, and T. Tsuda. 2002. "Responsibility and Cancer Disclosure in Japan." *Social Science and Medicine* 54: 281–293.

Feldman, E. 1985. "Medical Ethics the Japanese Way." *Hastings Center Report* (October): 21–24.

Fujiki, N., and D. Macer, eds. 1998. *Bioethics in Asia*. Christchurch, N.Z.: Eubios Ethics Institute.

Fukatsu, N., A. Akabayashi, and I. Kai. 1997. "The Current Status of Ethics Committees and Decision Making Procedures in General Hospitals in Japan." *Journal of Japan Association for Bioethics* 7: 130–136 (in Japanese).

Fukaura, A., H. Tazawa, H. Nakajima, and M. Adachi. 1995. "Do-not-Resuscitate Orders at a Teaching Hospital in Japan." *New England Journal of Medicine* 333: 805–808.

Hamano, K. 2003. "Should Euthanasia be Legalised in Japan? The Importance of Attitude towards Life." In *Bioethics in Asia in the 21st Century*, edited by S. Y. Song, Y. M. Koo, and D. R. J. Macer. Christchurch, N.Z.: Eubios Ethics Institute, pp. 110–117.

Hsin, D. H-C., and D. R. J. Macer. 2003. "Attitude towards Life and Death of Seniors in Taiwan." In *Bioethics in Asia in the 21st Century*, edited by S. Y. Song,

Y. M. Koo, and D. R. J. Macer. Christchurch, N.Z.: Eubios Ethics Institute, pp. 84–94.

Japan Medical Association. 1989. The Ministry of Health and Welfare and the Japan Medical Association, "Manual for Terminal Care of Cancer Patients." *Journal of the Japan Medical Association* 102 (suppl.) (in Japanese).

Kimura, R. 1995. "History of Medical Ethics: Contemporary Japan." In W. T. Reich, ed., *Encyclopedia of Bioethics*. New York: Simon and Schuster Macmillan, pp. 1496–1505.

Lock, M. 1995. "Contesting the Natural in Japan: Moral Dilemmas and Technologies of Dying." *Culture, Medicine and Psychiatry* 19: 1–38.

Lock, M. 2002. *Twice Dead: Organ Transplants and the Reinvention of Death*. Berkley: University of California Press.

Macer, D. 1992. "The 'Far East' of Biological Ethics." *Nature* 359: 770.

Macer, D. 1994a. *Bioethics for the People by the People*. Christchurch N.Z.: Eubios Ethics Institute.

Macer, D. 1994b. "Bioethics May Transform Public Policy in Japan." *Politics and the Life Sciences* 13: 89–90.

Macer, D. 1998. *Bioethics Is Love of Life*. Christchurch, N.Z.: Eubios Ethics Institute.

Macer, D. 1999. "Bioethics in and from Asia." *Journal of Medical Ethics* 25: 293–295.

Macer, D. 2001. "What Is Our Bioethics?" *Eubios Journal of Asian and International Bioethics* 11 (1): 1–2.

Macer, D. 2003. "Regional Perspectives in Bioethics: Japan." In *Annals of Bioethics*, edited by J. Peppin, Vol. 1 on Regional Perspectives.

Macer, D., T. Hosaka, Y. Niimura, and T. Umeno. 1996. "Attitudes of University Doctors to the Use of Advance Directives and Euthanasia in Japan." *Eubios Journal of Asian and International Bioethics* 6 (3): 62–69.

Maekawa, F., and D. Macer. 1999. "Japanese Concept of Family Privacy and Gentic Information." *Eubios Journal of Asian and International Bioethics* 9 (3): 66–69.

Morikawa, I. 1994. "Patient's Rights in Japan: Progress and Resistance." *Kennedy Institute of Ethics Journal* 4: 337–343.

Morioka, M. 2000. "Commentary on Tsuchiya." *Eubios Journal of Asian and International Bioethics* 6 (6): 180–181.

Morioka, M. 2001. "Reconsidering Brain Death: A Lesson from Japan's Fifteen Years of Experience." *Hastings Center Report* 31 (July): 41–46.

Nagoya High Court 1962, Decision 12.22.

Nie, J.-B. 2001. "Challenges of Japanese Doctor's Human Experimentation in China for East Asian and Chinese Bioethics." *Eubios Journal of Asian and International Bioethics* 11 (1): 3–7.

Rothenberg L. S., J. D. Merz, N. S. Wenge, M. Kagawa-Singer, D. R. J. Macer, N. Tanabe, S. Fukuhara, K. Kurokawa, H. L. Fuenzalida-Puelma, P. Figuueroa, J. G. Meran, E. Bernat, and T. Hosaka. 1996. "The Relationship of Clinical and Legal Perspectives Regarding Medical Treatment Decision-making in Four Cultures." *Annual Review of Law and Ethics* 4: 337–379.

Sakamoto, H. 1999. "Towards a New 'Global Bioethics.'" *Bioethics* 13 (4): 191–197.

Shinagawa, S. 2000. "Tradition, Ethics and Medicine in Japan." *Berliner Medizinethische Schriften*. Dortmund: Humanitas Publishing House, numbers 40/41.

Shirai, Y. 2003. "The Status of Ethics Committees in Japan." *Eubios Journal of Asian and International Bioethics* 13: 130–134.

Swinbanks, D. 1989. "Japanese Doctors Keep Quiet." *Nature* 339: 409.

Takeda, F. 1991. "Changing Attitudes towards Narcotic Use in Cancer Pain Management in Japan." *Postgraduate Medical Journal* 67 (suppl. 2): S31–34.

Tanida, N. 1991. "Patient's Rights in Japan." *Lancet* 337: 894.

Tokyo District Court 1971. Decision 5.19.

Tsuchiya, T. 2000. "Why Japanese Doctors Performed Human Experiments in China 1933–1945." *Eubios Journal of Asian and International Bioethics* 6 (6): 179–180.

Uemura, K. 2000. "A Position Statement by the Japan Geriatric Society for Terminal Care in the Elderly: A Draft of JGS Ethics Committee." *Journal of the Japan Geriatric Society* 37: 719–721.

Watts, J. 2000. "Japan Makes Older People Contribute towards their Health Care." *Lancet* 356: 2075.

Further updated references on bioethics in Japan can be found at the Eubios Ethics Institute World-Wide Web site: ⟨http://www.biol.tsukuba.ac.jp/~macer/index.html⟩.

8

End-of-Life Decision Making in Kenya

Angela Wasunna

End-of-life decision making in much of the developed world is associated with an aging population. As stated in the introduction to this book, most of the attention in the West has focused on the elderly as terminal patients. Much of the literature on death and dying is written with reference to this population. However, each year there are 56 million deaths in the world, 85 percent of which occur in developing countries (World Health Organization 2000a). For example, there are more than 40 million people currently living with HIV/AIDS, the majority of whom are in Africa and have little or no access to drugs (World Health Organization 2003). More than 8 million people contract tuberculosis each year, resulting in 2 million deaths, and 300–500 million cases of malaria result in 1 million deaths each year in the developing world (World Health Organization 1998). These potentially fatal infectious diseases affect all age groups in developing countries and raise complicated cultural, social, and economic end-of-life issues.

Having said that, an aging population is now a clear trend in the developing world. In Africa, for example, there are currently 38 million people over the age of 60. This number is projected to grow to 212 million by the year 2050 (HelpAge 2000). Steep declines in fertility throughout the continent will further increase the aging population.

In Kenya, 1999 population statistics revealed that there were 28,808,658 people living in the country. Out of this number, 788,631 were 65 years and above and fell under the United Nations' definition of the elderly. However, this interpretation is problematic because in much of Africa, including Kenya, the definition of "elderly" does not depend only on chronological age. Old age in many African countries is seen to begin at the point when active contribution is no longer possible. For others, the ages and number of children or grandchildren is an indicator of whether a person is considered elderly. Thus, socially constructed meanings of age are more relevant, particularly with regard to the roles assigned to older people (Heslop and Gorman 2002).

This chapter examines end-of-life decision making in Kenya from the perspective of the growing elderly population as well as a younger population that is succumbing to infectious diseases, particularly HIV/AIDS. It must be stated from the outset that there are currently almost no studies or data on the capacity to facilitate end-of-life decision making in Kenya, and indeed in much of sub-Saharan Africa.

Kenya's Health Care System

Like most former colonies, Kenya inherited a health care system at independence that was designed to provide care to a small fraction of the population; namely, the settler population, missionaries, and African workers in settler farms and establishments. During colonial rule, control of endemic diseases was the primary concern of the British regime. In 1963, when independence was obtained, Kenya had a three-tier health system in which the central government provided services at the district, provincial, and national levels; religious mission groups provided health care services at the subdistrict level; and the local government provided services in the major towns. In 1970, the government established a system of comprehensive rural health services focused on primary care and preventive medicine, with limited tertiary health care services.

Today, apart from health care services delivered by the government and religious organizations, nongovernmental organizations and private practitioners provide a wide range of services, from primary to tertiary care. The government's health care delivery system is still largely pyramidal, with national referral facilities at Kenyatta National Hospital and Eldoret Teaching Hospital at the peak, followed by provincial, district, and subdistrict hospitals, with health centers and dispensaries at the base (Kimalu 2001).

Between 1963 and 1991, infant mortality rates in Kenya dropped from 126 to 52 per 1,000 live births. In the same period, life expectancy rose from 40 to 60 years. The crude death rate dropped from 20 per 1,000 to 12 per 1,000 in 1993, and the crude birth rate from 50 per 1,000 to 46 per 1,000 over the same period. Immunization coverage rose to 76 percent in 1993 from less than 30 percent in 1963 (Government of Kenya 1999).

According to the Kenya Human Development Report of 1999, the positive gains Kenya achieved in reducing mortality rates between 1960 and 1992 have been reversed. For example, the infant mortality rate has increased from 51 in 1992 to 74 in 1998 per 1,000 live births. Immunization coverage has also declined from 79 percent in 1993 to 65 percent in 1998 (Kimalu 2001). One of the reasons for this reversal is that health care delivery in Kenya is severely underfunded. The public health expenditure is less than 5 percent of the annual gross domestic product (GDP), and the health expenditure as a portion of capital expenditure has declined from 5.54 percent in 1989 to 3.09 percent in 1996.

Structural adjustment programs mandated by the World Bank and the International Monetary Fund place more emphasis on curative care services, rather than on public health programs that are relatively cheap for users. As a result, there has been a general deterioration in the quality and quantity of health services and reduced access for the poor following the introduction of user fees. Declines in food availability as a result of prolonged droughts and increasing poverty have also acted to reverse the positive health trends.

The HIV/AIDS pandemic has also had profound negative effects on the health of the population. It has rapidly eroded the social and economic gains Kenya had achieved over the years, and it has also increased the cost of health care so that it is beyond the reach of most Kenyans. The total number of people infected with HIV in Kenya increased from 629,319 in 1992 to 1,506,000 in 1997. During the same period, the national rate increased from 7.4 to 11.8 percent, with the urban rate being higher than the rural rate (Government of Kenya 1999). Today, approximately 700 Kenyans die from AIDS each day (National AIDS Control Council of Kenya 2001).

It must be noted that alongside the government health care system, which basically provides Western medicine, traditional healers play a major role in providing health care services to Kenya's rural population.

In fact, in 1979, the government granted official recognition to traditional medicine by issuing a statement that read in part:

Traditional medicine and health care are an important part of the life of the people in the rural areas. However, more information is needed and will be collected ... with regard to both its substantive aspect and potential link with government institutions ... further, considerations will be given to the manpower aspects of the traditional sector, for instance, the extent to which certain cadres of selected traditional sector practitioners such as midwives, might be encouraged to serve in Government health institutions in the rural areas. (Republic of Kenya 1979: 136)

Although there are tensions between Western-trained doctors and traditional healers, the latter remain recognized stakeholders in Kenya's health care delivery system.

Having laid out the heath care delivery framework in Kenya, it becomes clear that the country is struggling to provide basic health care services to its citizens. Quality end-of-life care is defined by the U.S. National Academy of Sciences' Institute of Medicine (Field and Cassel 1997) as consisting of five elements, namely:

1. Overall quality of life
2. Physical well-being and functioning
3. Psychosocial well-being and functioning
4. Spiritual well-being
5. Patient perception of care

However, the provision of such care may not be a priority for the government of Kenya simply because it is overwhelmed with the health and other social needs of its population.

In trying to make a case for improving end-of-life care in poor countries, an important issue has to be addressed up front. Is it prudent to allocate the limited resources available to providing quality end-of-life care in developing countries when its populations are dying of diseases that could be easily prevented? Aren't the resources better spent on trying to improve people's lives rather than their deaths? In Kenya, as in most other African countries, most deaths do not take place in a hospital setting; rather, they occur in homes. Should the government, therefore, set up structures that may compete with this tradition, which arises not simply as a result of economic reasons but is also due to deep-seated customs and cultures?

In an article on care at the end of life, Peter Singer and Kerry Bowman confront this very question. They argue that both the lives and deaths of people in developing nations should matter; that it is not an either/or choice. They explain that if a person dies prematurely because of in-equalities in global health care, it is doubly unjust for that person to be condemned to an agonizing death. In addition, by focusing on improving end-of-life care, the groundwork may be laid for comprehensive, hu-mane, and ethical health care systems in developing countries (Singer and Bowman 2002). This is a persuasive argument. We should be concerned about how people live as well as how they die.

African customs and culture emphasize values such as dignity, honor, and respect both in life and death. Elaborate funeral rites in Kenya un-derline the importance of giving a person a dignified sendoff into the next world. Because life is considered a continuum that does not end at death, ensuring that a person moves into life's next phase in an honorable and decent manner is consistent with most African cultures.

What is the state of end-of-life care in Kenya today? The next sections briefly examine the major structures and/or factors that influence this care.

Health Services and End-of-Life Care for the Elderly

In order to have access to relatively good health care services in Kenya, one must have health insurance, which can be obtained through one's employer or bought through private health insurance companies. Wealthy Kenyans are able to enroll in insurance plans or pay for health care expenses themselves, but for the majority of Kenyans, such services are out of their reach.

The government has also set up a national health insurance scheme known as the National Hospital Insurance Fund, in which each working Kenyan is required by law to pay a certain percentage of his or her in-come toward this fund. The government then subsidizes the contributor's health care costs in both private and public institutions, depending on the level of contribution. It should be noted that the subsidies provided by the government are usually inadequate and patients must usually use their own funds as a supplement to pay the treatment costs. The government also has a national social security scheme that is supposed to provide pension and other social benefits to persons who have retired from government employ.

Clearly, if one is not wealthy, or has never worked in the public sector, and/or is at present unemployed, there are only limited options available for financing health care. Unfortunately, a great majority of the elderly population in Kenya fall into this bracket and/or work in the informal sector. Despite their advancing age, they continue to support their families by caring for children, managing the home, and taking part in agricultural work. Older people also make valuable contributions to society as custodians of traditions and cultural values that are passed on from generation to generation. Unfortunately, their economic contributions are usually unpaid and unrecognized, but nevertheless form an indispensable part of development (HelpAge 2000).

With the present cost-sharing regimes in most public hospitals, the elderly find it almost impossible to obtain specialized health care services or obtain pain-relieving drugs. In addition, the government does not have any special geriatric programs to cater to the health needs of the growing elderly population, although there are a few such programs run by nongovernmental organizations. This is despite the fact that in many areas where HIV/AIDS has ravaged the community, the elderly are performing parenting and caregiving duties for their sick children as well as their grandchildren. Their own health is vital to the health of others in the community.

A recent survey in Africa by HelpAge International found that there are almost no programs initiated by African governments that allow older people to receive free medical services. Furthermore, most elderly people, particularly in rural areas, do not even have transport money to take them to health centers to seek treatment. In addition, older people are routinely excluded from primary health education systems (HelpAge 2000). Unfortunately, Kenya's elderly are sometimes reluctant to use health facilities because they feel that they are using resources that are best left for the young, who still have their lives ahead of them. Thus the picture is quite bleak in terms of formal health care services for the elderly population. The extended family support system and traditional healing services, with their more holistic approach, however, have ameliorated some of the adverse effects caused by a lack of formal health facilities.

Health Practitioners and Medical Technology

As stated earlier, most deaths in Kenya do not occur in hospitals. Furthermore, preventable infectious diseases primarily cause these deaths. According to the World Health Organization, the five leading causes of death in sub-Saharan Africa are HIV/AIDS, acute lower respiratory infections, malaria, diarrheal diseases, and measles (World Health Organization 2000b).

For those deaths that do occur in hospitals, what type of end-of-life care is available? Are there doctors and other health care personnel who are trained in palliative medicine? Again, no studies have been carried out to determine the capacity of Kenyan hospitals to deliver quality end-of-life care. Outside of the hospice movement, there are almost no health care personnel with specialized palliative experience.

Kenya has an acute shortage of medical personnel. In 1965 the country had 710 trained doctors, 26 dentists, and 148 pharmacists. By 1996, the number of health staff had increased to 3,971 doctors, 685 dentists, and 1,147 pharmacists (Government of Kenya 1999). However, 80 percent of the doctors and dentists work in urban areas, which have only 20 percent of the population (Kimalu 2001).

Medical universities in Kenya often do not include geriatric training in their curricula. This has led to the nondevelopment of geriatric medicine as a specialized field. There is an acute need to train nurses and other health care officers in palliative medicine as a distinct field. The curative model taught in Kenya's medical schools focuses on treatment and prolonging life. Death and dying issues are not given much prominence. This needs to change, particularly given the sheer numbers of people dying in the country in all age groups.

Lifesaving medical technologies can only be found in the large hospitals in Nairobi, Mombasa, and Kisumu (the three largest cities in Kenya).

The demand for this equipment far outstrips the supply. Decisions as to who gets on the lifesaving machines are usually determined by cost. Only the very rich (or those with good insurance coverage) can pay for the machines and these are almost always allocated on a first-come basis. Hospital administrators have a lot of power in deciding who gets on the machines, and there is little room for ethical review of their decisions. There are no current statistics on the costs of dying (in a hospital setting), partly because the cost varies greatly from one hospital to another. However, it is not unusual for medical costs to be as much as $10,000 for persons who have been on lifesaving machines in private hospitals.

The Legal System

The practice of medicine in Kenya is highly paternalistic. Doctors are regarded very highly and patients usually defer decision making to their physicians. However, doctors are governed by a number of laws and ethical rules. Laws pertaining to medical practice can be found in the Kenyan Constitution, Statutes (Acts of Parliament), By-laws, Common Law, and Ethical Codes.

Euthanasia is illegal. A physician who actively participates in any form of mercy killing is guilty of a criminal offense and can be punished under the penal code (Chapter 63 of the Laws of Kenya). It is also considered an unethical practice under the Kenya Medical Practitioners and Dentists Board's Code of Ethics. Such a doctor is subject to disciplinary proceedings by the Medical Board, which can result in the loss or suspension of his or her practicing certificate.

One of the weaknesses in Kenyan health law is the definition of "death." The law is gray in this area. A doctor is allowed to remove patients from lifesaving machines after he has pronounced them "clinically dead." The problem is that Kenyan law defines a person as "clinically dead" only after his or her heart has stopped beating, and not when a person has suffered brain death. If a person's heart is still beating, even though the brain is clinically dead, the law still considers the patient alive, and any attempt by the doctor or the patient's family to remove the person from the lifesaving machine constitutes euthanasia, a criminal offense. Furthermore, organs cannot be harvested from a person who is brain dead but whose heart is still beating because of the definition of death as set out in Kenyan law (Human Tissue Act, Chapter 252, Laws of Kenya).

Under contract law and common law, advance directives are permissible. However, they are seldom used, for a variety of reasons. First, under common law, once a person has been pronounced clinically dead, they do not have property rights to their own bodies. Therefore a person can state how he or she would like their body treated upon death or how they should die (as long as such directives are within the limits of the law), but a judge or executor of the estate is not bound by law to honor those wishes if there are other overriding interests.

Furthermore, in many African cultures, writing advance directives or wills can be interpreted to mean that one is "inviting death." It is not culturally appropriate to anticipate death by putting down in writing how one wants to die or what should happen to one's property in death. Many Kenyans refrain from writing legal wills for this very reason. It is unlikely that this culture will change in the near future. Moreover, the role of the family is important in Kenyan culture. Family members are considered to have the best interests of their fellow members at heart. Consequently, many people defer decision making to family members rather than putting their wishes in written form.

Finally, there has not been much education about advance directives. Most lawyers do not know how to draft advance directives or how to educate their clients about the process. Furthermore, in a society in which doctors are highly paternalistic, not many people are willing to go against their physician's professional advice and determine their own destinies. This will change slowly as Kenyans become more and more aware of their health rights.

In terms of decision making, Kenyans, like many other Africans on the continent, live in close kinship systems in which extended family members are virtually indistinguishable from the nuclear family. In end-of-life situations, which family members, then, should be legally able make decisions on behalf of the patient if he or she does not have the capacity to do so? The law is not specific on this question; however, under common law, spouses can make decisions for each other, as can parents for minors. In the case of minors (under the age of 21), if the parents or legal guardians of the child cannot be located during an emergency, the clinical head of the institute may give the necessary consent. In the case of minors in institutions (juvenile remand homes or approved schools), the manager of such an institution may, on the advice of a medical officer, make medical decisions on behalf of the minor. The High Court of Kenya, however, is the legally mandated guardian of minors in Kenya and, upon application, it can overturn any decision made on behalf of a minor under the "best interests" standard.

In emergency cases, where an adult's life is in danger and a life or death decision has to be made immediately, the law allows medical personnel to provide treatment to the patient as long as (1) the patient has not been able to communicate his or her wishes; (2) the treatment is not against the patient's will; and (3) the treatment is in the patient's best interests. In the case of the mentally ill who are incapable of making decisions, the Mental Health Act, Chapter 248 of the Laws of Kenya provides that the husband, wife, or another relative may make decisions on behalf of the patient. If there is no such person available, surrogate decision powers fall to any other person who submits a written application to the court explaining why they should make such decisions on behalf of the patient (typically this is the head of the institution or doctor in charge).

The Effect of HIV/AIDS on End-of-Life Care

HIV/AIDS is the single most devastating issue facing much of the developing world today. Africa has 10 percent of the world's population and 63 percent of the world's HIV cases. An average of 3,800 adults in Africa are infected daily. AIDS has lowered the average life expectancy by as much as 17 years in some countries. Prime-aged, skilled, and productive adults are leaving behind parents and children who are expected to cope emotionally and economically with the loss of family members. Unfortunately, few studies have examined the effects of the AIDS epidemic on the elderly in developing countries.

The elderly in Kenya are generally affected by HIV/AIDS in a variety of ways. For example, they are left to care for young and parentless children, and they also become caregivers for their sick children. Second, the use of the elderly in market and nonmarket activities has been affected because they spend more time caring for their families (Dayton and Ainsworth 2002). After the death of a child, the elderly adult may have to increase participation in earning activities to replace the earnings of the deceased individual (Barnett and Blaikie 1992).

Health professionals and health service planners have routinely neglected the considerable impact of the AIDS epidemic on older people in terms of the risks they themselves face from HIV infection. According to a HelpAge report, distorted views are partly to blame for this. For example, the assumption that HIV/AIDS is a disease of only the younger generation has led to the impression that older people do not contract the virus (Okatcha 1999). It is thought that they are least likely to contract HIV/AIDS, so that the symptoms, which resemble those of other ailments, are sometimes undetected or are wrongly diagnosed under the general category of "normal old age diseases" (Okatcha 1999)

Older people in Kenya are in fact silent sufferers of HIV/AIDS. The virus does not differentiate among ages, and older people contract the disease through sexual intercourse with infected persons, through the use of unsterilized medical equipment, or through contaminated blood products and fluids. In terms of policy making, therefore, there is a huge gap in the provision of counseling and other health services to older HIV/AIDS sufferers.

It is imperative that the elderly be included in HIV/AIDS counseling, prevention, and treatment programs, particularly given the new roles they have to play as caregivers in their families. Whereas HIV/AIDS in Kenya mostly affects those between the ages of 15 and 45, it also affects the elderly, and this needs to be underscored to policy makers, who have perennially ignored this population in important health and support programs.

HIV/AIDS has had severe impacts on the younger, economically productive population. As stated previously, it is putting a disproportionate caretaking burden on families. Most Africans describe their families as including extended family members, and traditionally children are expected to care for their parents in their old age. The loss of people in the younger age group has serious economic repercussions on family life because the most vulnerable, those under 18 and the elderly, are left without the income they provide.

Euthanasia is slowly gaining prominence owing to the devastating effects of this disease. Many younger HIV-infected people do not want to burden their elderly parents or relatives by making them take care of them as well as the children they leave behind. In some cases, an HIV/AIDS diagnosis creates a feeling of complete hopelessness in many people because without good health insurance or personal funds, there are not many health options available to the patient. The temptation to end one's life and avoid putting the burden of caretaking on the family can be quite strong. There has thus been a surge of requests for assisted suicide among infected patients. This puts an emotional burden on doctors, who from a legal point of view cannot participate in any form of mercy killing, yet understand the situation faced by their patients.

Requests for euthanasia have also been made on the legitimate grounds of pain and suffering. Because palliative care in Kenya is not readily available, persons suffering from the end stages of AIDS may want to end their lives in order to put an end to the suffering and indignity caused by the disease. In the absence of treatment and pain-alleviating medication and in the context of severe poverty and despair, death is often seen as the only option available to end suffering. These are all issues that need to be addressed openly by the medical and legal community as well as by health policy makers and the public at large.

The Hospice Movement in Kenya

Despite the lack of health services, infrastructure, and personnel to effect quality end-of-life care in Kenya, there is a beacon of hope in the form of the hospice movement. This movement is defying all the odds and providing quality end-of-life care to suffering patients. Excluding South Africa, Kenya's hospice was the second one to be set up in sub-Saharan Africa. The first one was set up in Zimbabwe and it initially served the white community exclusively and was focused on cancer patients. An English woman named Ruth Woolridge founded Nairobi's hospice in 1991. It was radically different from its Zimbabwean counterpart in the sense that it was set up to meet the needs of the local Kenyan population. The hospice is funded largely by a charitable foundation in the United Kingdom called Hospice Africa, but it also receives sponsorship and enjoys support from the local community.

Hospice Africa has opened other hospices in smaller towns in Kenya like Nyeri, Mombasa, Eldoret, and Meru. These hospices are directed toward the care and counseling of persons who are terminally ill with cancer and other incurable diseases. They offer counseling services to the patients' families and friends and provide education and training services in palliative care. Hospice Africa has thus been instrumental in developing palliative care services in Kenya. It has supported doctors' and nurses' salaries at the hospices, and provided vehicles and medicines and other overheads to support the centers in Kenya.

Hospice Africa in Kenya makes treatment available to people for pain relief and symptom control. Unlike the hospices of other African countries, those in Kenya, Uganda, and Zimbabwe provide morphine to patients through their respective governments. In addition, Hospice Africa integrates traditional medicine and healing practices into their own practice. Traditional healers are affordable, and they offer a holistic and spiritual approach to death and dying. They are routinely invited to participate in teaching sessions where they share their own knowledge in palliative care with other heath care workers.

In 2002, Hospice Africa's Kenyan Chapter set up a diploma program in palliative care in conjunction with Oxford Brookes University in the United Kingdom. This collaborative venture offers practitioners from Africa the opportunity to achieve an internationally respected qualification with minimum absence from their own practice and workplace setting (Hospice Care Kenya 2002).

Although Hospice Africa in Nairobi initially catered primarily to cancer patients, the high mortality from HIV/AIDS has shifted the patients it now serves from cancer patients to those with HIV/AIDS. Because many HIV-infected people cannot afford treatment for opportunistic infections, HIV is seen as a terminal disease, and patients come to the hospices when they are in severe pain. Twenty-five to 50 percent of patients with full-blown AIDS require pain control medication. In Kenya, only a registered physician can prescribe morphine and other controlled pain medication. Unfortunately because of the acute shortage of doctors, it is difficult to ensure that all AIDS patients in need of pain medication will have access to such treatment in the public health care system.

Conclusions

Even without the HIV/AIDS epidemic, Kenya is barely coping with the burden of diseases like malaria, tuberculosis, and diarrheal diseases. The Ministry of Health has an acute shortage of health care personnel and service infrastructure. There is, however, much that can be done to improve end-of-life care. As argued, because death in Kenya is really a public health problem, given the sheer numbers dying, the government has a moral obligation to ensure that its citizens do not die agonizing deaths and thus suffer doubly.

Kenya needs to embark on education programs to inform the public, policy makers, the private sector, and legislators that it is possible to reduce the impact of HIV/AIDS and other terminal illnesses by providing palliative care. Palliative drugs are much cheaper to provide and easier to manage than medication for treating HIV/AIDS, and as the government tries to find creative ways to provide this treatment, it should also take into account providing pain-relieving medication. There are many people who would be productive members of society if they had access to such medication. The elderly, particularly those who have added responsibilities that are due to the AIDS burden, would benefit immensely from such programs while they are caring for their own families.

In this regard, organizations like Hospice Kenya, health nongovernmental organizations, medical schools, and the Ministry of Health need to network with each other and build links so that they work together to promote the provision of palliative care. Hospice Uganda, for example, is partnering with the Ugandan Ministry of Health and bringing all the aspects of palliative care into the country's national health plan.

In addition, the legal community needs to revise its present laws to bring them up to date with the realities. For example, perhaps in view of the lack of doctors, senior health officers should be allowed to prescribe pain medication in public hospitals under the supervision of doctors. Furthermore, the use of advance directives could be couched in a culturally sensitive manner to allow provisions for community decision making in end-of-life situations. There is an obvious need for more research on death and dying in Kenya. In order to have effective national policies on end-of-life care, it is critical to have more information on what the current quality of care is and how improvements can be measured.

Perhaps most important, there should be a focus on home-based palliative care. As emphasized, most Kenyans die at home, and they are usually buried at their ancestral homes. Most of them still have extended family members who care for them. This existing infrastructure could be harnessed to provide effective palliative care. Hospice Uganda, for example, has satellite centers that send doctors and nurses into villages to follow up patients and provide them with palliative drugs and care in the comfort of their homes. Relatives of the patients are also involved in the treatment and care of their loved ones. Another African example is the Chikankata hospital in Zambia. This hospital provides both hospital care and intensive follow-up of terminally ill patients through community-based workers who go to see patients in their homes and who also give basic palliative care training to family members.

Traditional healers can provide important leadership in these kinds of initiatives because they are generally familiar with the community and are well respected. They should be integrated into the mainstream health care system and their expertise used to the advantage of those in need.

The challenges in providing end-of-life care in Kenya are many; however, there are already success stories in other parts of the developing world that can be emulated. It cannot be overemphasized that given the number of deaths occurring in the country each day, this is an area that can no longer be ignored and one that is deserving of national attention and urgent action.

References

Barnett, T., and P. Blaikie. 1992. *AIDS in Africa: Its Present and Future Impact.* London: Belhaven Press.

Dayton, J., and M. Ainsworth. 2002. *The Elderly and AIDS: Coping Strategies and Health Consequences in Rural Tanzania.* Working Paper 160. Cited on a Web page of the Population Council. Africa. www.popcouncil.org/publications/wp/prd/rdwplist.html (visited on September 7, 2002).

Field, M. J., and C. Cassel, eds. 1997. *Approaching Death: Improving Care at the End of Life.* Washington, D.C.: National Academy Press.

Government of Kenya, 1999. *Kenya Human Development Report.* Nairobi: Government Printer.

HelpAge. 2000. *Ageing Issues in Africa: A Summary.* Nairobi: HelpAge International.

Heslop, A., and M. Gorman. 2002. *Chronic Poverty and Older People in the Developing World.* CPRC Working Paper 10. Nairobi: HelpAge International.

Hospice Care Kenya. 2002. *Annual Report and Accounts: 1 April 2001–21 March 2002.* Bristol, United Kingdom: Hospice Africa.

Kimalu, P. K. 2001. "Debt Relief and Health Care in Kenya. Kenya Institute for Public Policy Research and Analysis (KIPPRA)." Paper presented at a conference on Debt Relief and Poverty Reduction, UNU/WIDER, Helsinki, Finland, August 17–18, 2001.

National AIDS Control Council. 2000. *The Kenya National HIV/AIDS Strategic Plan 2000–2005.* Office of the President, Nairobi: Reprographics Press.

Okatcha, K. 1999. "Old AIDS on older people." *Courier* 176: 62.

Republic of Kenya. 1979. *Development Plan 1979–1983.* Nairobi: Government Printer.

Singer P., and K. Bowman. 2002. "Quality care at the end of life." *British Medical Journal* 324: 1291–1292.

World Health Organization. 1998. Fact Sheet 203. Cited on a Web page of the World Health Organization. www.who.int/inf/inf-fs/en/fact203.html (visited on September 7, 2002).

World Health Organization. 2000a. Fact Sheet 104. Cited on a Web page of the World Health Organization. www.who.into.inf-fs/en/fact104.html (visited on September 7, 2002).

World Health Organization. 2000b. Fact Sheet: Backgrounder. Cited on a Web page of the World Health Organization. www.who.int/inf-fs/en/back001.html (visited on September 7, 2002).

World Health Organization. 2003. "Global AIDS Epidemic Shows no Sign of Abating." http://www.who.int/mediacentre/releases/2003/prunaids/en/print.html (visited December 3, 2003).

9

End-of-Life Decision Making in the Netherlands

Henk ten Have

The Dutch End-of-Life Debate

During the past three decades, the debate concerning end-of-life decision making in the Netherlands has been dominated by the issue of euthanasia. The debate often starts with so-called "paradigmatic cases" that appear to call for euthanasia. These cases are exposed in the popular and scientific literature to illustrate the relevance and plausibility of euthanasia in particular circumstances. They also present a popular and frightening image of the end of life. However, as the debate has developed over time, more and more cases have surfaced that differ significantly from these paradigmatic cases, suggesting that euthanasia might also be justified in other conditions and circumstances. Thus we find that the euthanasia debate has gradually expanded from its clearly delineated early stage to a much broader practice.

In the Netherlands, after three decades of debate and practical experience, euthanasia still is not an established or normal practice. A new law, implemented in April 2002, makes euthanasia a legitimized medical intervention under particular conditions. However, the legal regulation of euthanasia does not mean that the practice has lost its controversial and contentious character. While the Dutch Parliament was debating the new bill, the "Brongersma case" added new dimensions and created confusion. How could simply being old, without physical and mental illness but tired of life, be a condition of unbearable suffering? Mr. Brongersma was 86 years old and had no physical or mental ailments, but was tired of living; in his view, life had become unbearable and an unacceptable source of suffering. And then came the case of Wilfred van Oijen, the general practitioner who had figured prominently in the well-known Dutch television documentary, "Death on Request." He was on trial because he had terminated the life of a nursing home patient at the request of the family rather than the patient; van Oijen was found guilty of "murder" yet not punished because he acted "with integrity."

The situation in regard to euthanasia, therefore, remains complex and multifarious. Opponents of euthanasia point to the expansion of the practice. They also argue that the focus on euthanasia ignores the wide variety of approaches to end-of-life care that are available in other countries. Advocates do not think that this expansion is necessarily problematic but cannot agree on where to draw the line between acceptable and unacceptable cases. The only thing that most people seem to agree about is that the current practice has certain drawbacks that need to be amended, including the notification of euthanasia cases and the provision of alternatives such as better palliative care.

Policies for Euthanasia and Assisted Suicide

The new legislation in the Netherlands (Termination of Life on Request and Assisted Suicide Act) essentially does three things. First, it revises Articles 293 and 294 in the penal code. Second, it stipulates the requirements of due care that the physician must abide by in order to be immune against punishment. Third, it delineates the process for reporting and evaluating euthanasia cases.

Legalization

The old Article 293, which prohibits murder at the victim's request, has become the first paragraph of the new Article 293. A second paragraph has been added that legalizes euthanasia performed by physicians. In an attempt to counter criticism from abroad, the Dutch government has insisted that the new law does not legalize euthanasia. After all, Article 293, § 1 of the penal code still prohibits any and all forms of requested murder. Paragraph 2 merely provides a punishment exclusion ground for euthanasia, akin to the more generic exclusion ground included in Article 40 (force majeure). At the same time, under the new law, the physician who commits euthanasia in accordance with the requirements of due care will never be in contact with the legal authorities. He or she has to submit a report to the municipal coroner, which is reviewed by a special committee. If the report is accepted by the committee, the case will not be advanced to the prosecutor and no legal proceeding will ensue. The same is true for the physician who assists in a patient's suicide. The old Article 294 prohibiting such assistance has remained in force, but physicians are excluded if they fulfill the requirements of due care.

Requirements of Due Care

In addition to revising the criminal law, the new law also provides detailed guidelines for the practice of euthanasia. In fact, these guidelines are not very new. The various court decisions in the 1980s had already resulted in a variety of guidelines. In 1987, a bill was proposed that reduced the punishment for requested murder to $4\frac{1}{2}$ years, specified that good palliative care should not be considered requested murder even if death ensued, and provided a list of requirements of due care. The law did not pass. But in 1990, the Ministry of Justice went ahead and issued a similar list of requirements as part of a formal notification procedure. Since euthanasia was a crime, one could not legally expect physicians to notify the authorities of their actions. No suspect is legally required to assist in his or her own conviction. But without notification, it would also be impossible to regulate the practice. In 1993, Parliament decided in favor of a typically Dutch maneuver: formally issue guidelines on how to commit a crime and then report it to the authorities. The new law incorporates these guidelines and the notification procedure from 1993.

The law states that the "requirements of due care" that the euthanizing physician must fulfill in order to be immune from punishment are as follows. The physician must (1) hold the conviction that the request by the patient is voluntary, well-considered and lasting, and that the patient's suffering is without prospect of relief and unbearable; (2) inform the patient about his or her situation as well as about the prognosis; (3) believe, together with the patient, that there is no reasonable alternative solution for the patient's situation; (4) consult at least one other independent physician who has seen the patient and formed an opinion about these requirements of due care; and (5) terminate the patient's life with due medical care. In short, the new law does not set any new, stricter, or even more precise requirements of due care for the practice of euthanasia. It does, however, create two new expansions of the already widespread practice of euthanasia.

First, it specifically states that a person does not need to be competent when euthanized (Article 2, §2). The patient can make a request for euthanasia in writing in advance of becoming incompetent, a kind of "living will for euthanasia." The law thus inherits all the problems that living wills typically invoke: Consider, for example, a patient in the beginning stages of Alzheimer's disease. She fears a downhill slope and writes a living will requesting euthanasia. Can this patient, who has never before been demented and does not know how her brain, mind, and attitudes will be affected by the disease, accurately predict that her wish for euthanasia will be lasting and is the only reasonable alternative, as stipulated by requirements (1) and (3)?

More troublesome is the fact that minors can request euthanasia as well. The law stipulates that a minor between the ages of 16 and 18 who appears mature can be euthanized at his or her request, provided the parents have been consulted (Article 2, §3). Note that the parents cannot stop the euthanasia. In fact, they may not be able to stop the euthanasia of their 12-year-old child either. If the parents of a child between the ages of 12 and 16 oppose euthanasia, but the physician believes that "serious harm" can be prevented by means of euthanasia, the physician can override the parents and euthanize the 12-year-old at the child's request (Article 2, §4).

Notification and Evaluation

The third and largest part of the new law delineates the procedure for notification and, foremost, evaluation of euthanasia. Since the Law on Burial and Cremation already contains guidelines specifying how a physician should notify the authorities when she or he has committed euthanasia, the new law only had to formalize the evaluative process.

As before, the physician is legally required to inform the coroner that the patient did not die of natural causes, but as a result of either euthanasia or assisted suicide. Simultaneously, the documents are forwarded to one of the regional committees that have been formed to evaluate all reported euthanasia cases. Each of these committees consists of at least three members—a lawyer who serves as president, a physician, and an ethicist or moral theologian. These committees evaluate whether the physician committed euthanasia in accordance with the requirements of due care. A simple majority of votes is decisive. If the physician's act is approved by the committee, the physician will be informed in writing, but no report will be sent to the legal authorities. Only if the committee finds that the physician has not acted properly will the regional prosecutor be informed.

The evaluation of euthanasia is completely retrospective. In fact, Article 16 specifically prohibits any member of these committees from providing prospective advice to physicians who are planning to euthanize one of their patients. This is remarkable since euthanasia is now legal. While it was illegal, the authorities evidently could not evaluate and approve euthanasia prospectively. The courts could only find, in hindsight, that the physician had been compelled to euthanize the patient because of force majeure. But now that euthanasia has become legal, it is not clear why the tradition of retrospective evaluation has been continued.

It should be pointed out that at present there are only five regional committees. At the current reporting rates of approximately 2,000 cases per year, this means that each committee must review 400 cases a year, or about 8 cases each week. Since these committees operate only 1 day a week, they have about 1 hour to review each case. This makes it clear that it would be impossible for the committee to carefully examine each case in depth and determine that the patient was truly competent, informed, and not pressured by family members or health care providers; that the request for euthanasia was sincere, authentic, and not in fact a desperate call for compassion and help; that the patient's condition was beyond prospect of relief and all alternatives of good end-of-life care and symptom relief were exhausted; and that the patient's suffering was truly unbearable and lasting. All of this needs to be assessed and evaluated, as well as the manner in which the physician went about euthanizing the patient—and all in about an hour or less.

The Practice of End-of-Life Decision Making

Although active euthanasia has always been a criminal offense, in the past three decades medical specialists and general practitioners have been quite open about their euthanasia practice, publishing case reports in influential Dutch medical journals. This professional candor has coincided with (and probably was fostered by) a considerable judicial lenience toward physicians practicing euthanasia under strict conditions. Yet, in spite of this professional openness and legal lenience, many physicians who perform euthanasia were not prepared to face the risk of the legal consequences of their practice and as a result completed death certificates incorrectly. Consequently, the overall incidence of active euthanasia in medical practice remained unknown, although estimates varied from 2,000 to 20,000 per year.

In January 1990, the "Remmelink committee," composed of three lawyers and three physicians, was established to obtain an empirical understanding of the frequency and nature of euthanasia in medical practice. A random population of some 400 physicians were interviewed about their past experiences and asked to provide (anonymously) the true cause of death of each of their patients expected to die in the next 6 months. Finally, an attempt was made to verify the cause of death in a random sample of some 8,500 recent deaths. In September 1991, the committee issued its report (Commissie Onderzoek Medische Praktijk inzake Euthanasie 1991). This policy decision to survey and analyze empirical data has been important for two reasons—first because the focus of scientific study was wide, taking into consideration end-of-life decision making in general, and second because once the research pattern was set, the studies have been replicated so that comparative data are now available for 1990, 1995, and 2001.

According to this study, physicians made decisions on the deaths of their patients in approximately 44 percent of all patients who died in 2001 (van der Wal et al. 2003). These decisions included whether to discontinue life support, provide increasing doses of pain medication, withhold treatment, assist in suicide, or commit euthanasia. Assisting in suicide in 1990 was found to occur in some 400 cases a year. Remarkably, in 2001 this number decreased to 300 cases. Euthanasia, "intentionally ending life," was practiced some 2,300 times (1.9 percent of the total mortality in 1990). During the past decade, the number of euthanasia cases has increased to 3,500 (2.2 percent of total mortality in 2001). Unexpectedly, it was also found that in 1990 there were, 1,000 cases of termination of life without explicit request; in 2001 this was 900 cases. In euthanasia or assisted-suicide cases, 77 percent of the patients suffered from malignant neoplasms. Medical doctors were asked to rate the suffering of the last patient they had euthanized as well as to assess the patient's life expectancy. According to the respondents, 93 percent of these patients showed severe physical suffering. In 13 percent of the cases, life expectancy at the moment of execution of the request was estimated as more than 1 month; in 41 percent it was less than 4 weeks but more than 1 week; in 36 percent, less than 1 week; and in 10 percent less than a day (van der Wal et al. 2003). The quantitative data of the various surveys are reproduced in table 9.1 (van der Wal and van der Maas 1996; van der Maas et al. 1996; van der Wal et al. 1996, 2003).

The main objective of the legislation is to allow better public control of the practice of euthanasia. The law, however, does not define it or clarify in which cases euthanasia is legal. One criticism of the law is that it does not make any distinction between termination of life at the request of the patient and that done without explicit request. Both conditions

Table 9.1
End-of-life decisions in the Netherlands, 1990–2000

	1990	1994	2001
Deaths in the Netherlands	128,824	135,675	140,377
Requests for euthanasia			
later in the disease	25,100	34,500	34,700
explicit	8,900	9,700	9,700
Euthanasia	2,300	3,200	3,500
Assisted suicide	400	400	300
Life termination without explicit request	1,000	900	900
Withholding or withdrawing treatment	22,500	27,300	28,360
with the explicit intention to shorten life	11,594	17,637	18,249
Termination because of intensification of pain and symptom management	22,500	20,000	28,215
also with the intention to shorten life	5,150	4,070	2,800

have to be reported. However, it is obvious that exemption from prosecution is only given if the requirements of due care have been met. Another criticism is the paradoxical nature of the legislation. Since termination of life is formally a crime, physicians who break the criminal law are obliged by the new law to report unlawful activities and to provide evidence that might lead to their prosecution. However, the law apparently does not achieve its objective. The 1995 survey shows that the majority of physicians (59 percent) do not report life-terminating acts. Also in 2001, with the system of review committees already functioning, 46 percent of cases were not reported.

It is difficult to conclude from the empirical findings that euthanasia in the Netherlands is less frequent than assumed by protagonists and antagonists. One problem is that such conclusions fail to take into account the fact that many physicians do not interpret and classify their actions as euthanasia even when they strictly fall under the range of the definition; that is, an active medical intervention to intentionally terminate life at the explicit request of the patient (Gunning 1991; ten Have and Welie 1992). For example, the survey data reveal that hastening death was the explicit intention of the administration of high doses of "pain" medication in at least some of the cases in which potentially lethal analgesics were administered (1 and 1.5 percent of all deaths in 1990 and 1995, respectively). And, in an additional 5.2 percent (1990) and 2.1 percent (1995), death was at least partly intended. Thus, there is no case for indirect effect because death was the intended, direct effect. Also in cases of withholding and withdrawing life-sustaining treatment (including tube feeding), it was the explicit intention to shorten life in 9 percent of all deaths in 1990, and in 13 percent of all deaths in 1995 and 2001 (van der Wal et al. 2003).

Van Delden and colleagues (1993a) have argued that the formulation of the intention (i.e., hastening death) seems to be the same in these cases as in euthanasia proper, but that the "sameness" of the intentions can be questioned. They claim that intentions ultimately are private and therefore beyond public evaluation. It may be agreed that in many cases it is very difficult to prove the intentions of the physician who hastens death, but this is primarily a lawyers' problem. Moreover, the intention of the actor has been made an essential element in the official definition of euthanasia, and even in the legal definition, despite the foreseeable difficulties in proving the physician's intentions. The point is that if the intention to terminate the life of the patient is definitive for euthanasia, the number of cases in the Netherlands is considerably higher than the "official" Dutch definition of euthanasia.

Another difficulty with the interpretation of the medical practice of euthanasia is whether or not there is a slippery slope. From the surveys, one could conclude that within a short 5-year period (1990 to 1995) the number of requests for euthanasia and the requests granted increased; requests alone increased by 37 percent. It is also obvious that for an increased number of patients, requesting euthanasia is normal behavior and is seen as a kind of guarantee against suffering that is made early in the disease process. At the same time, it is remarkable that during the last period (1995 to 2001) the number of euthanasia cases increased only slightly, while the number of euthanasia requests has stabilized.

Furthermore, a majority of Dutch physicians have been personally involved in life-terminating acts (in 2001, 57 percent of all physicians and 71 percent of all general practitioners). Nonetheless, the 2001 survey also showed that only 54 percent of cases were reported. Also, consultation with a colleague (one of the formal conditions for permissible euthanasia) did not occur in 25 percent of cases. These facts, combined with the substantial number of life-terminating actions carried out without explicit request, have led some authors to the conclusion that the Dutch practice is sliding down a slippery slope (Hendin 1997; Jochemsen and Keown 1999). Other commentators argue that it is not (Angell 1996).

An unexpected finding, given the inclusion of an explicit request in the "official" definition of euthanasia, was the number of cases in which there was no explicit request by the patient. The surveys show about 900 patients whose death was caused or hastened by physicians without an explicit request. This number pertains to patients who although no longer competent to make decisions, apparently suffered severely, and does not include cases where medically futile treatments were withheld or withdrawn. Although it is not clear how many of these cases were involuntary (i.e., if they were able to communicate, the patients would have expressed the wish not to be euthanasized), the absence of an expressed request precludes qualifying these cases as euthanasia proper. Nonetheless, the Remmelink committee felt that these cases of non-voluntary termination of life should not be of concern, but should be thought of as "providing assistance to the dying." Nonvoluntary termination of life was justified because the suffering of those patients had become "unbearable." Death would have occurred quickly anyway (usually within a week) if the physician had not acted. Elsewhere, the committee adds that actively ending life when "the vital functions have started failing," is "indisputably normal medical practice" (Commissie Onderzoek Medische Praktijk inzake Euthanasie 1991, p. 15).

Although they are evidently not compatible with the requirements of the new legislation, there is an increasing tendency to justify such cases. In 24 percent of these cases, although an explicit request was absent, there had been "some deliberation" with the patient. Already in 1991, it was clear that although about a quarter of these 1,000 patients had previously expressed the wish to die, this was not always the leading rationale for the physicians euthanizing them. Only 17 percent of the physicians involved in these cases mentioned the "previously uttered request of the patient" as their reason for terminating their patients' life. The researchers explained this discrepancy by arguing that physicians more often are guided by their own "empathy" with the patient's unspoken but probable wishes, than by explicit oral or written patient requests (Commissie Onderzoek Medische Praktijk inzake Euthanasie 1991: 51).

This explanation indicates a significant shift in moral justification. Respect for autonomy had always been the prime argument in favor of active euthanasia. But now that quite a number of cases occur without an explicit request by a patient, other arguments are brought forward to defend this practice. Thus, a paradox emerges between this line of reasoning and the opposing reasoning of the original advocates of voluntary euthanasia that suffering is a purely subjective phenomenon. Consequently, only the patient can decide whether his or her suffering has become unbearable, and thus termination of life is only justifiable when the patient so requests. It seems that some advocates of euthanasia use the latter strategy when defending the right of the competent patient to autonomously opt for euthanasia and the former strategy when defending the practice of euthanasia on the mentally incompetent patient. A similar ambiguity is shown in van der Wal's study (1992). His conclusion that the majority of euthanized patients have severe physical and emotional suffering does not follow. It merely can be concluded that the physicians in retrospect think this about their patients.

What the medical practice of euthanasia in the Netherlands reveals is that the ethical justification has been shifting from respect for autonomy to relief of suffering. This has created a conflict within the strategies for justifying euthanasia. The two arguments are mutually exclusive. It only makes sense to talk about respect for autonomy if a physician refrains from making judgments about the patient's benefits. It is logically impossible to base a euthanasia decision on both autonomy and beneficence (van Delden et al. 1993b). Moreover, the primacy of the bioethical principle of respect for patient autonomy has always been grounded in the presumed inability, or virtual inability, of physicians (or any other third persons) to make reliable judgments about a patient's well-being or suffering.

If, on the other hand, physicians are now considered to be well able to make such judgments, the decisive factor is no longer the patient's explicit request for euthanasia, but the concurrence of the physician with the patient's assessment of the suffering being unbearable. The physician will comply with the "autonomous" request of the patient only if he or she agrees that the patient's suffering is, indeed, unbearable or the quality of the patient's life is so poor that the patient is better off dead. In fact, the patient's request will only be regarded as an autonomous request if it is rational from a medical point of view. In this line of reasoning, nothing changes when the same medical rationality indicates that euthanasia is appropriate but the patient is no longer capable of communicating. When the patient is incompetent or his or her views are unavailable, the physician is still capable of making the assessment.

Both empirical research and political debate reveal that in daily practice two moral considerations compete with each other: respect for autonomy and relief from suffering. From the physician's point of view, the latter consideration appears to be the most important; it is the prime motive for performing euthanasia in cases of incompetent patients who, in the judgment of the physicians, suffer unbearably. It is also a strong motive in cases of competent patients since less than a third of all requests are fulfilled. This emphasis on suffering as the predominant moral justification could have been expected from the history of euthanasia since the term derives from the Greek for "good" or "merciful" death. Definitions of euthanasia often refer to suffering from incurable diseases as the fundamental condition. It is also argued that the crucial difference between euthanasia and murder is the motive; murder would be killing for reasons other than kindness (Thomasma and Graber 1990). The history of euthanasia primarily is the history of "mercy killing." It is the argument of compassion, not the argument of respect for autonomy, which has been the most basic moral justification for euthanasia (Meerman 1991).

This observation implies that the outcome of the euthanasia debate is paradoxical. Physicians now seem to have ultimate control over the moral justification of active euthanasia. If the life of a patient is terminated because the physician feels morally justified on the basis of the unbearable suffering of the patient, it is difficult to distinguish the compassionate involvement of the doctor from paternalism. The doctor is not wicked or criminal; he or she has the best possible motives and offers the most compassionate care available, but yet, this is paternalistic behavior. The doctor knows best when it is your time to die. Intervention-driven medical technology led to the euthanasia movement in the first place, but there is no sign that this characteristic of medicine has significantly changed. What was the initial cause of the problem is now considered the prime solution to it (ten Have 1998).

Approaches to Death and Dying

As noted earlier, the paradigm case that is typically presented in debates of euthanasia depicts a competent patient in the final stages of life with an incurable disease and in a state of unbearable suffering. Once becoming terminal, the patient himself or herself issues a voluntary and persistent request for euthanasia. The various elements of this paradigm case have been incorporated in the official Dutch definition of euthanasia. This definition emphasizes the intentional ending of the life of a patient by a physician at the specific request of that patient. Indeed, the label "passive euthanasia" is no longer used, because the types of decisions this label refers to do not involve the physician's intent to end the patient's life and are therefore not considered euthanasia proper. Likewise, cases where there is no patient request are not considered cases of euthanasia.

Controlled Death

Both the structure of the paradigm case and the official Dutch definition of euthanasia exemplify the significance of one specific moral justification of euthanasia, that is, the moral principle of respect for individual autonomy. This principle is thought to provide the proper counterbalance against medical power. And although individual freedom is not as decisive a political principle as it is in the United States, Dutch people harbor strong libertarian sentiments that favor an almost absolute right to respect a patient's autonomy.

The significance of autonomy has given rise to a specific approach to death and dying. Death is considered a personal decision, not an event that befalls human beings and needs to be accepted as part of life. The autonomous individual determines when and how death will occur. It is the rational outcome of an assessment of one's life, the secularized last judgment made by a person. According to this image of controlled death, the duty of the physician is to ascertain whether the patient has made a voluntary and carefully considered decision.

However, on closer inspection it is all but clear that the concept of patient autonomy is significant in the practice of euthanasia. Advocates of euthanasia argue that autonomy implies the possibility and justifiability of making decisions about one's own life, including ending it, but this proposition appears at odds with the philosophical and political tradition out of which the notion of respect for individual autonomy grew. In this libertarian tradition, autonomy has been deemed a basic characteristic of a human being precisely because it guarantees that each person is free and able to make decisions according to his or her own free will. Nevertheless, it is questionable whether an appeal to individual autonomy can justify ending one's life. If autonomy is a basic value, can a person eliminate the very basis of this important characteristic? If this is true, the implication is that there are certain limits to autonomy, even when arguing within the confines of a philosophy of autonomy itself.

Even if we assume that people have the right to end their lives, a second question immediately emerges. Is it morally justifiable for other people to assist in this? In short, even if suicide is morally justifiable, that does not mean assisting in suicide is too. In the Netherlands, it is generally assumed that assisting in suicide is justifiable, particularly if it is done by a physician. Why a physician? This again is not self-evident because in other domains of life we actually prohibit physicians ending the lives of other people. Although the Netherlands does not have the death penalty, almost everybody seems to agree that of all people, physicians should not be engaged in capital punishment. There is no logical connection between the morality of suicide and that of a physician ending the life of a patient. If it is the moral principle of autonomy that justifies suicide, one can consistently argue only that the doctor may prescribe the drugs necessary for the patient to end his or her own life, so that in the end, the moral responsibility remains in the hands of the patient. Yet euthanasia is much more popular in the Netherlands than physician-assisted suicide.

Preemptive Death

The image of controlled death and the primacy of the principle of autonomy, although important in the early stages of the euthanasia debate, has become less influential because of the emergence of the image of preemptive death. Today in the public debate, the prominent image is that of a fast and painless departure from life. The Protestant ethicist Harry Kuitert has made a comparison between living and being in a room; one enters through one door and can leave through another. This image of a sudden departure coincides with the expectation that suffering will be superfluous and preventable; a good death is one where the person still is active and feels well, just prior to any deterioration and decline that are due to disease or aging. If unbearable suffering is a major justification for euthanasia, why wait until the suffering has become unbearable?

Research data for 1995 and 2001 show that compared with an earlier study from 1990, the number of requests for euthanasia has grown (van der Wal et al. 2003). A distinction is made between two types of patient requests. The first is a request to have euthanasia "in due course." For example, when patients are first diagnosed with cancer, many want to find out about their physician's stance toward euthanasia, and they do so by asking for euthanasia. In 2001, more than 34,000 patients made this type of request (compared with 25,100 in 1990). It is important to attend to the meaning of these requests to have euthanasia in the longer term. Such requests do not necessarily mean that these patients want to die. These patients are not dying, but are in the initial stages of a potentially lethal disease. They are anxious and concerned that at a later stage when they are suffering the doctor will do his or her utmost to relieve that suffering. A request for euthanasia is a quite effective way to ensure the complete attention of health care professionals.

The second type is a request for euthanasia "in the foreseeable future." This is a specific request when the patient is at the stage where death is imminent. In 2001, there were 9,700 of these requests for euthanasia (compared with 8,900 in 1990). These requests involve more deliberation than the requests of the "in due course" type because a practical decision on whether to grant or refuse the patient's request must be made. In 2001, of those 9,700 requests, 3,500 were granted (compared with 2,300 out of 8,900 in 1990) (van der Wal et al. 2003).

A striking conclusion can be drawn from the research data. Only a minority of euthanasia requests are actually carried out. Two-thirds of the requests for euthanasia are not granted. Apparently the patient's own explicit and persistent request is not decisive. This conclusion is supported by another set of data collected by the same research team. These data show that there were 4,700 cases of active termination of life in 2001. Of these 4,700 cases, 900 (or 19 percent) were without the patient's request. These 900 cases do not qualify as euthanasia proper (as delineated in the standard definition), indicating that there is a considerable practice of termination of life without the explicit request of the patient.

These findings raise serious doubts about the value of the respect-for-autonomy argument within the practice of medicine. For medical doctors, respect for autonomy is not the decisive motive for action. In daily practice, the most important consideration and the main moral justification for euthanasia is relief of suffering. It is not really relevant whether the patient requests euthanasia or not. If in their physicians' opinion, patients are not suffering unbearably or their suffering can be treated, their request for euthanasia will not be granted. If, on the other hand, the doctor estimates that the situation of unbearable suffering is worse than being dead, he or she will consider the option of active termination of treatment. In such dire circumstances, the patient's request is not even a necessary condition. Data reveal that many physicians simply assume that patients would have wanted euthanasia even if the patients have not been articulate in requesting it or have merely hinted at the possibility of euthanasia, as well as if the patients are incompetent, psychiatric patients, demented elderly, or handicapped newborns.

These data raise the question of what really is the basic justification for euthanasia. It is evident from a historical perspective that euthanasia has never been primarily linked to the issue of autonomy. It was primarily considered a form of mercy killing, an act of compassion where killing the person was better than letting him or her suffer. In the present Dutch debate, two different sets of moral justifications appear to be operative which are, moreover, often at odds with each other: a nonmedical justification that emphasizes respect for patient autonomy (and the importance of a voluntary request), and a medical justification that emphasizes relief of suffering (and the importance of a situation of unbearable suffering). The paradox of the Dutch euthanasia debate is that it started out as a protest against medical power, emphasizing patient autonomy as a counterbalance, but 30 years later, the power of physicians has only increased because it is physicians who decide whether the patient's suffering is so unbearable that the request for euthanasia can be granted (ten Have 2001).

This paradox is fueled by the highly problematic consequences that either alternative would bring forth. For example, if autonomy were truly decisive, ending human life without an explicit request would have to be ruled out. On the other hand, all patient requests for euthanasia would have to be taken seriously. The number of euthanasia cases would be at least three times the present number. Stringent rules and guidelines would have to be put in place to make sure that the patients' requests are reliable (e.g., repeated request, second opinion, documentation). But the grounds for the request can no longer be evaluated; they are the proper domain of the individual patient's valuation. All of this appears quite consistent, but as the recent case of Mr. Brongersma shows, the consequences of this logic are very troublesome. In December 2002, the Supreme Court of the Netherlands rejected being tired of life as a justification for euthanasia; there had to be some kind of medical condition explaining the suffering of the patient.

If, on the other hand, the decisive factor is relief of suffering, the discretionary power shifts to the physician, who has to decide whether the patient's suffering is unbearable and whether euthanasia is therefore justified even if the patient does not (or cannot) request it. Now the question arises of what are objective criteria that allow a physician to judge whether the patient's suffering is indeed unbearable. Without such criteria, decision making will depend on the subjective and arbitrary values of individual physicians.

The emerging image of preemptive death is useful to mitigate the tensions between medical power and patient autonomy. The patient still has some control over the moment of death if there is some underlying medical condition. In deliberation with his physician, he or she can conclude that death is desirable as a preemptive strike against the terrors of dying. It is reminiscent of the aphorism of Epicurus: death is not the enemy but rather suffering is. Rational human beings anticipate future suffering and possible deterioration. Medical professionals should support advance care planning and assist in determining the appropriate moment of a preemptive action.

The studies reviewed here provide useful data about the reasons for euthanasia requests and illustrate the emergence of this new image of death and dying. As would be expected, "unbearable suffering" is frequently mentioned, as are "dehumanizing condition," "loss of dignity," and "pain." Considerably more surprising is a cluster of reasons that concern the individual patient's ability to cope with the situation: "meaningless suffering," "dependence," and "tired of life." These reflect the expansion of suffering as a justification for euthanasia from the somatic suffering of the paradigmatic cancer patient to mental and even spiritual suffering. Most remarkable is a third category of reasons, such as "escape from deterioration of suffering," "prevention of suffocation," and "prevention of pain." These reasons show that euthanasia is no longer considered only an escape from unbearable suffering, but also a sensible strategy to prevent such a state from occurring in the first place. Why wait until the suffering is becoming unbearable? The popularity of this new approach to euthanasia is evidenced by the fact that the Dutch minister of health herself suggested during the parliamentary debates on euthanasia that it would be wise for people in the early stages of dementia to draft an advance directive requesting euthanasia. She also advocated the distribution of suicide pills among the elderly.

Palliated Death

Reflecting upon these data, the question arises of whether the Dutch focus on euthanasia, emerging as an option in the search for a good death, has not at the same time reduced the range of care options available at the end of life. If euthanasia becomes a means of preventing suffering altogether instead of the last resort when all alternatives to relieve suffering have failed, there is no longer a need for alternative means of pain relief. Why develop therapies to ameliorate pain and suffering when euthanasia can prevent the emergence of severe suffering altogether? Why should society create social structures and networks to involve the elderly in human interaction and social life when euthanasia is an adequate remedy for older persons like Mr. Brongersma who experience loss of meaning in life? We thus find that the emphasis on euthanasia tends to deflect attention from other approaches to good death and dying. This finding is supported by 41 percent of the physicians interviewed in the 2001 euthanasia survey (van der Wal et al. 2003).

For example, many hospitals in the Netherlands only recently developed policies for withholding and withdrawing treatment. Expert centers in pain control and management have been established only in the past decade. Contrary to other countries, palliative care has become a target of Dutch health policy only in the past few years. Only recently has there been a move toward the development of a wider range of available options at the end of life, options through which many requests for euthanasia could be prevented. The question is whether this is not too little too late.

Paradoxically, the commitment to a good death created the euthanasia movement and in turn the commitment to euthanasia reduced the number of options available to patients to bring about a good death. Only recently has interest in palliative care started increasing. Euthanasia consultants in particular are increasingly aware of the wide range of possibilities for ameliorating suffering developed in the new discipline of palliative care. This new awareness is creating another, new, image of death and dying, "palliated" death. A death can be a good death, not because it is fully controlled by the patient, or is a timely escape from the growing burden of suffering, but because it is the appropriate last chapter of the personal biography, always difficult and burdensome, but tolerable and worthwhile. However, medical professionals should be able to provide the best expertise available to make the quality of this last part of life as comfortable as possible. The recent debate on terminal sedation demonstrates the emergence of this new image of palliated death. Putting terminal patients to sleep has always been rejected because of the implied loss of control and autonomy. Today, the option of sedation is being discussed more and more and explored by many health care professionals.

Conclusions

The Dutch experience with euthanasia shows that it is imperative to make a distinction between three ethically different conditions:

1. *Withholding or withdrawing life-sustaining treatment.* In these cases, the treatment is ended and the patient can die. It is not the doctor who is the cause of death, but the underlying disease or condition of the patient. Setting limits to medical interventions can help to prevent situations where patients can only die by asking the doctor to end their lives or to assist in causing death. In many countries, the bioethical debate is now very much focused on decisions not to treat. Many hospitals, for example, are developing policies for not resuscitating patients in certain conditions. Better palliative care and pain management, as other alternatives

for euthanasia, are also now receiving much attention in many European countries.

2. *Active termination of life at the request of the patient.* Debates over the past three decades have been focused almost exclusively on this situation. The basic moral question is whether individual persons should be allowed to end their own lives. If this basic question is answered positively, the next question is whether another human being can assist in ending this life. In the discussion, it is generally assumed that only a physician can do so, but it is unclear what the implications are for medical practice in general. If a doctor can end a human life, medicine will have completely new goals of executing the wishes of autonomous persons (being a kind of service on request), fighting suffering even if it means killing the sufferer (being a kind of ultimate care), or both.

A more fundamental philosophical concern has to do with the ideal of total self-control that shows itself in practices of managing mortality. The idea of a human being as *causa sui*, producing his or her individual well-being and being in control of his or her life and existence, negates the finiteness of human beings. Moral debates on euthanasia revive a very old ideal, defended for example by Pelagius (fifth century A.D.), that the powers of a human being suffice for achieving one's own perfection, and also that since perfection is possible for human beings, it is obligatory. However, in Western culture these perfectionist ideals have always been criticized and relativized (from St. Augustine onward) as a denial of human frailty and a refusal to accept that human life in principle is uncontrollable and beyond personal autonomy.

3. *Active termination of life without the request of the patient.* In this situation, relief of suffering is regarded as the primary goal of medicine. It is evident, however, that what is regarded as suffering implies a subjective judgment. Physicians are no better equipped than other persons to accept or disqualify various conditions of suffering; their judgments about which suffering is unbearable may therefore vary widely. In this situation, one may also fear a diminishing acceptability of various conditions (for example, in the case of handicapped newborns or demented elderly) within society at large.

The evolution of the euthanasia debate in the Netherlands also provides some lessons that can be significant for debates concerning euthanasia in other countries that are considering legalization of euthanasia and physician-assisted suicide.

• Notwithstanding the fact that the Dutch euthanasia movement originated out of a concern for the medicalization of death and dying, euthanasia and assisted suicide have become medical practices and are the prerogative of physicians.

• Even though human dying and death will always defy human control, there appears to be an incessant attempt on the part of contemporary societies and modern medicine in particular to control death. This explains the attractiveness of euthanasia and physician-assisted suicide in the Netherlands, as opposed to palliative medicine and hospice care.

• The increasing focus on the patients' quality of life is an opportunity for the emerging approach of "palliated death," going beyond the images of "controlled death" and "preemptive death."

• The ethics of end-of-life care is complex, and careful distinctions are necessary to identify care approaches that make the last phase of human life worthwhile and at the same time mitigate the harmful effects of medical interventions, without having recourse to euthanasia in order to effectuate the desire for a good death.

• The Dutch experiment shows that preventing the practice of euthanasia is both an important and a feasible alternative. If euthanasia is truly to be a means of last resort, manifold other strategies toward good end-of-life care have to be realized first, including improved palliative care units and consultation services, expanded home-care services and hospice care options, and revisions of medical education as well as patient education programs.

References

Angell, M. 1999. "Euthanasia in the Netherlands—Good News or Bad?" *New England Journal of Medicine* 335 (22): 1676–1678.

Commissie Onderzoek Medische Praktijk inzake Euthanasie. 1991. *Medische beslissingen rond het levenseinde*. Gravenhage: Staatsdrukkerij's.

Delden, J. J. M. van, L. Pijnenborg, and P. J. van der Maas. 1993a. "Dances with Data." *Bioethics* 7 (4): 323–329.

Delden, J. J. M. van, J. Pijnenborg, and P. J. van der Maas. 1993b. "The Remmelink Study. Two Years Later." *Hastings Center Report* 23 (6): 24–27.

Gunning, K. F. 1991. "Euthanasia." *Lancet* 338: 1010.

Have, H. A. M. J. ten, 1998. "Euthanasia and the Power of Medicine." In *Asking to Die: Inside the Dutch Debate about Euthanasia*, edited by D. C. Thomasma, T. K. Kushner, and C. Ciesielski-Carlacci. Dordrecht: Kluwer, pp. 205–220.

Have, H. A. M. J. ten, 2001. "Euthanasia. Moral Paradoxes." *Palliative Medicine* 15: 505–511.

Have, H. A. M. J. ten, and J. V. M. Welie. 1992. "Euthanasia: Normal Medical Practice?" *Hastings Center Report* 22 (2): 34–38.

Hendin, H. 1997. *Seduced by Death: Doctors, Patients and the Dutch Cure.* New York: W.W. Norton.

Jochemsen, H., and J. Keown. 1999. "Voluntary Euthanasia under Control? Further Empirical Evidence from the Netherlands." *Journal of Medical Ethics* 25: 16–21.

Maas, P. J. van der, G. van der Wal, I. Haverkate, C. L. M. de Graaff, J. G. C. Kester, B. D. Onwuteaka-Philipsen, A. van der Heide, J. M. Bosma, and D. L. Willems. 1996. "Euthanasia, Physician-assisted Suicide, and Other Medical Practices Involving the End of Life in the Netherlands, 1990–1995." *New England Journal of Medicine* 335 (22): 1699–1705.

Meerman, D. 1991. Goed doen door dood maken. *Een analyse van de morele argumentatie in vijf maatschappelijke debatten over euthanasie Tussen 1870 en 1940 in Engeland en Duitsland.* Kampen: J. H. Kok.

Thomasma, D. C., and G. C. Graber. 1990. *Euthanasia: Toward an Ethical Social Policy.* New York: Continuum.

Wal, G. van der. 1992. *Euthanasie en Hulp bij Zelfdoding Door Huisartsen.* Rotterdam: WYT Uitgeefgroep.

Wal, G. van der, and P. J. van der Maas. 1996. *Euthanasie en Andere Medische Beslissingen Rond het Levenseinde.* The Hague: SDU Uitgevers.

Wal, G. van der, P. J. van der Maas, J. M. Bosma, C. L. M. de Graaff, B. D. Onwuteaka-Philipsen, D. L. Willems, I. Haverkate, A. van der Heide, J. G. C. Kester, and P. J. Kostense. 1996. "Evaluation of the Notification Procedure for Physician-assisted Death in the Netherlands." *New England Journal of Medicine* 335 (22): 1706–1711.

Wal, G. van der, A. van der Heide, B. D. Onwuteaka-Philipsen, and P. J. van der Maas. 2003. *Medische Besluitvorming aan het Einde van het Leven. De Praktijk en de Toetsingsprocedure Euthanasie.* Utrecht: De Tijdstroom.

10

End-of-Life Decision Making in Taiwan

Tai-Yuan Chiu

Hospice and palliative care are widely recognized in Taiwan as the ideal model of care at the end of life. Since the number of terminal cancer patients and the medical expenditure for the end-of-life services in Taiwan have increased in recent years, palliative care has been advocated as a moral responsibility of medical professionals. The hospice movement in Taiwan includes the following milestones. The first inpatient hospice care unit was established in 1990; the Natural Death Act (*An Ling Huan He Yi Liao Tiao Li*) was enacted in 2000, and the National Health Insurance (NHI) Benefit Payment began in 2000. The Board of Hospice and Palliative Medicine has been certifying physicians as specialists in palliative medicine since 2000, and the governmental noncancer patient project was expanded in 2002.

Currently in Taiwan, there are 29 inpatient care units, providing 418 hospice beds, and 40 home-care programs. Empowered by several medical professional groups and fully supported by the government, the hospice movement has gained momentum in Taiwan. Despite that, hospice care covered only 16.3 percent of the 32,993 patients who died from cancer in 2001 (Lai 2003).

Estimated Costs of Dying

Taiwan's national health insurance provides comprehensive health care services. NHI expenditure in 1999 grew by 30 percent over 1996, or a total of US$9 billion (Department of Health 2002), prompting increased efforts to contain costs. The cost of treating the terminally ill is sometimes blamed for the steady increase in health care costs because of the intensive and technically complex medical treatment employed during the last stages of life, although it appears that many of these treatments are futile and unnecessary (Scitovsky 1994). Many international studies indicate that patients who die use more medical resources and have higher medical expenses than patients without a fatal prognosis (Ginzberg 1980; Zweifel et al. 1999). This situation has been referred to as "the high cost of dying" (Ginzberg 1980: 308).

Chen (1998) analyzed the last-year-of-life costs in the second half of 1996 in Taiwan. The results show that 0.1 percent of all beneficiaries used 5.4 percent of the total of inpatient expenses paid by the Bureau of National Health Insurance (BNHI) in the last year of life. Moreover he found that 67 percent of the total cost of inpatient hospital care was spent during the last month prior to death (Chen 1998). However, Chen's study recorded only hospital care expenses. In Liu and Yang's study (2002), the total NHI expenditure in the last year of life for the 9,369 deceased (7.8 percent of total deaths) in 1999 was US$71.6 million. About 54 percent of all medical expenses in the last year of life were incurred in the last 3 months of life. Nephritis and cancer were the most costly causes of death, with per capita expenses of US$15,220 and US$10,828, respectively (Liu and Yang 2002).

Places for Dying

In Taiwan, the ongoing trend is that an increasing number of people die in hospitals. This phenomenon has been observed over the past several decades. In the year 2000, in Taiwan about 35 percent of the 124,481 total deaths took place in hospitals and 58 percent of the deaths occurred at home. In 1991, hospital and home deaths accounted for 30 and 58 percent, respectively, and in 1984, those figures were 24 and 62 percent, respectively (Department of Health 1975, 1992). Actually, in many cases dying patients were only kept breathing through a manual ventilator, so as to go home and die a "home death," as Taiwanese traditional culture demands.

On the other hand, according to the survey conducted by the Taiwan Academy of Hospice Palliative Medicine, only about 3,000 people (8.4

percent of the total of cancer deaths) died in a hospice in 2000. However, would this be a situation that Taiwanese people want? Chiu's studies show that the preferable place of death for Taiwanese is at home (80 percent among those in a rural community, 70 percent in urban communities) (Chiu and Ohi 1995; Chiu 1997a). When asked to give reasons for going home to die, most of the Taiwanese indicated that their home is their familial place (79.6 percent) and the majority also pointed out that they would wish to be surrounded by their family at death (56.7 percent). The rationale for choosing to stay in a hospital was that they did not wish to be "an additional burden to the family" (100 percent), rather than because they would expect to have better medical treatment (26 percent).

Therapeutic Strategies and Advance Directives in Terminal Illness

Determining a therapeutic strategy is usually a difficult clinical decision, especially in the area of terminal illness. Chiu et al. (2000b) found that on admission 15 percent of terminal patients in Taiwanese hospices insisted on being cured as the goal of treatment. However, by the fifth week in hospice, all had changed their perspective regarding this goal. Nevertheless, frustration with this issue appeared again in the following week, demonstrating a fluctuation in the acceptance of the goal of treatment. Regarding advance directives, Hu et al. (2001) found that almost every medical professional in charge of caring for terminal cancer patients had obtained written informed consent when forgoing cardiopulmonary resuscitation (CPR). However, in less than half of the cases (47 percent), had doctors obtained informed consent from both patients and the family. In 53 percent of cases of forgoing CPR, only a proxy family consent was obtained. One study regarding advance directives for the preferred therapeutic strategy at the terminal stage indicates that the majority of Taiwanese residents expressed a desire to use advance directives for the preferred therapeutic strategy (90 percent). However, the preferred mode of communication was to give the directive orally (69 percent) rather than as a written document (21 percent) (Chiu and Ohi 1995).

Cancer Pain Management and Opioid Availability

Cancer has been the leading cause of death in Taiwan since 1982. Pain is one of the major problems faced by cancer patients. More than 36 percent of newly diagnosed Taiwanese cancer patients and 85 percent of patients in hospices reported pain problems (Ger et al. 1998; Chiu 1997b). The high incidence of cancer pain is an important issue and may indicate inadequate pain control in Taiwan. Inadequate education about pain control, misunderstandings about morphine tolerance, and concerns about the side effects of opioids have been raised by Taiwanese physicians and nurses. Chiu's 1997 survey on the use of analgesics for cancer pain shows that only one-third of primary care physicians acknowledged that the regular use of morphine was appropriate in the control of moderate and severe pain from cancer (Chiu 1997b). On the other hand, about one-third of these physicians mistakenly approved the occasional use of meperidine and analgesics.

In regard to patients' perspectives, social and cultural influences on the use of opioids should be considered. Pain is more likely to be endured in cultures where stoicism is valued, or when the expression of feelings is not encouraged, such as in a Taiwanese culture influenced by Confucian thought. Because of these beliefs, Taiwanese patients avoid taking, or reduce their dose, of pain medication. Studies in Taiwan have shown that cancer patients believe that enduring pain is necessary (Lin and Ward 1995). Taiwanese health care providers might also expect patients to endure pain.

In the study by Chiu and colleagues, opioid use is one of the major ethical dilemmas in palliative care (Chiu et al. 2000b). Perhaps because of the widespread misunderstanding of the medical role of opium-derived compounds as a result of the opium wars in China in 1840, some patients and families still prefer to tolerate pain rather than use morphine. Another important factor affecting pain control is the use of herbal drugs in accordance with Taiwanese beliefs, which, as many patients fear, might have adverse interactions with Western medication.

As to national narcotics policy, in 1995 the Taiwanese government examined national drug control policies to determine if there were overly restrictive provisions that would impede the prescribing or dispensing of narcotic drugs needed for medical treatment of patients. It explored their availability and distribution for such purposes and made the necessary adjustments. Currently, Taiwanese national drug control policy recognizes narcotics as being absolutely necessary for the relief of pain and suffering. It establishes the government's obligation to make adequate provisions to ensure the availability of narcotics for medical and scientific purposes, including the relief of pain and suffering. The government has also established an administrative authority for implementing this obligation, including licensing, estimates, and statistics of narcotics use.

Actually, the government, with the cooperation of several health care professional groups, including the Taiwan Hospice Organization and the Taiwan Academy of Hospice Palliative Medicine (TΛHPM, *An Ling Huan He Yi Xue Xue Hui*), has identified and addressed concerns of health care professionals in prescribing opioids. Furthermore, the government has informed health professionals about the legal requirements for the use of narcotic drugs by providing many opportunities to discuss mutual concerns. Chiu's (2003) survey of cancer care professionals in Taiwan shows that only 14 percent of the total respondents still usually have trouble deciding whether to prescribe morphine. Currently, the deficiencies of opioid availability for the relief of pain and suffering include inadequate modes of opium-derivative medications, myths about morphine and addiction among patients and families, limitation of opioids to large urban centers, and lack of access in rural areas. In Taiwan, the only opioids available are codeine, tramadol, the Fentanyl patch (25, 50, 75 mg/h dosages), and morphine (tablet, syrup, parenteral use). Rotation of opioid drugs is inconvenient in clinical practice in the current situation.

End-of-Life Decision Making

It is a very difficult issue for terminal patients and their families to change the goal of treatment from "cure" to promoting "better quality of life." Even among cancer care professionals, there is an ethical dilemma in telling the truth about a terminal condition. Hence many patients with terminal cancer receive anticancer treatment until the last moment of life. That is the reason patients referred to hospice care have an average survival time of only 3 weeks (Chiu et al. 2000a). That is a very limited time for hospice and palliative care professionals to provide active, comprehensive care for the relief of all suffering or to achieve the best quality of life. The causes of late referral, which are common in Taiwan, might be inadequate education of the population about life and death, poor knowledge and skills in truth telling, lack of palliative care training, etc. Furthermore, a study investigating family-related barriers to truthfulness in cases of terminal cancer found that families felt it would be "unnecessary to tell aged patients the truth" (Hu et al. 2002: 486). The families always request that medical professionals not disclose the truth about the diagnosis and prognosis of cancer to aged patients. This situation makes the aged patients unable to participate in numerous decisions about plans for treatment and care or to exercise their right to choose, which inevitably affects the quality of care. The issues mentioned here are going to be among the future priorities of the hospice and palliative care movement in Taiwan.

It is worth mentioning that age is a significant factor in decisions to choose a therapeutic strategy for end-of-life care. The proportions of primary tumors found in hospice patients mirrored the overall cancer mortality in Taiwan, except for liver cancer, which in a study showed a lower rate than that in the general population of Taiwan (10.8 versus 20.4 percent). It is believed that the relatively young age of liver cancer patients may have influenced the decision of these patients to choose palliative care (Chiu et al. 2000a). Otherwise, few hemato-oncological patients were admitted to hospices (Chiu et al. 2000a), perhaps because of ethical difficulties in justifying the indications for blood transfusion.

Regarding the general public, Chiu's studies in 1993 and 1997 found that the majority of residents in both rural and urban areas expressed their willingness to choose promotion of life quality (72 to 75 percent) rather than prolongation of life (27 to 30 percent) if they had a terminal disease (Chiu and Ohi 1995; Chiu et al. 2000b). However, their real decisions differ significantly when the same people face the choice of therapeutic strategy for family members such as their parents or children. In the case of children with cancer, the parents' decisions always focus on prolonging life rather than promoting the best quality of life for their children. Family members frequently ask medical professionals to do their best to prolong the life of the patients who are their loved ones.

This conflict also occurs commonly in truth telling. In Confucian culture it is common practice not to disclose the truth about an illness, especially to a terminal cancer patient, on the basis of nonmaleficence. This mutual pretense prevails because both sides are unwilling to hurt each other and do not know how to communicate with each other. Many decisions are made only by the families and medical professionals; only one-quarter of the patients admitted to a hospice understand their terminal condition and the purposes of palliative care. The mutual pretense occurred in half of the admitted patients. One-quarter of the patients did not even know that their condition was terminal (Yao et al. 1997). In this circumstance, some important clinical decisions, such as sedating therapy for refractory symptoms, morphine use for dyspnea control, and do-not-resuscitate orders are chiefly made only by the families and medical professionals (Chiu et al. 2001).

Natural Death Act in Taiwan: Legislation to Reduce Unwanted Suffering

The Natural Death Act was approved on May 26, 2000. This is an important issue for about a hundred thousand terminally ill patients in Taiwan and their families, and for professionals as well. It aims to restore dignity of life for those who are suffering from a hopeless terminal illness. It took 6 years for this act to be passed. Early in 1994, many hospice promoters called for attention to the quality of life and the right to a good death for terminally ill patients. During the 6 years before passage, many opinions were voiced by different parts of society—some persons even called for euthanasia—which made the process of establishing this act an obstacle course. Euthanasia (*anlesi*) is intended to shorten a patient's life and relieve the sufferings of patients and families; thus it conflicts with the principles of palliative care. Euthanasia is not approved in Taiwan either by law, by religion, by ethics, or by culture.

After numerous debates, sessions, and negotiations with members of the legislative committee, the Natural Death Act was finally passed by the Legislative Yuan on the third reading. The birth of this act came rather late compared with some Western countries; however, it has been the first one for an Asia-Pacific country. Under legal protection, patients are now able to live and rest in peace. With the passage of this act, health professionals will be able to create high standards for quality of life in hospice care, and unnecessary medical expenses can be avoided.

This act consists of fifteen regulations. It states clearly that terminally ill patients have the right to make a will choosing hospice palliative care, either wholly or partially, or to create a durable power of attorney, and appoint a person to sign a will on behalf of the patient when he or she is unable to express his or her own will freely. This act also gives the patient the right to withdraw the signed document. Patients under 20 years must have a legal representative. Those who do not want to be resuscitated must have two doctors certify that they suffer from a terminal illness, and there needs to be two witnesses (who cannot be health professionals) to the signing of the will.

Since passage of this act, therefore, patients can now obtain for themselves the right to a good death. This act is to be extensively promulgated to the public. The Bureau of Medical Affairs of the Department of Health prepares consent forms and the procedural details. Some hospice-promoting organizations have conducted numerous promotional and educational activities on will preparation and signing to ensure that the spirit of this act can be put into operation.

On November 11, 2002, the Legislative Yuan passed the Natural Death Act Revised Rules (*An Ling Huan He Yi Liao Tiao Li*) in response to problems in implementing the earlier act. Although patients did sign the consent forms, things often became more complicated than doctors in end-of-life care had envisaged. For example, when terminally ill patients experienced the growing complications of their disease, they were unable to express their will or to act for themselves. Under this sort of pressure, family members were often puzzled and usually delivered the patient to the emergency room of a hospital, but in many cases family members did not bring the patients' consent forms with them. Also, since it is often a matter of life or death, it is common practice for emergency room doctors to conduct "first aid" using medical life-support systems if there is no informed consent from the patient. Once the patient's condition was stabilized, family members usually recalled that the patient had previously expressed the willingness to forgo cardiopulmonary resuscitation, or families acknowledged that cardiopulmonary resuscitation would only make the patient suffer. The discouraging result, however, was that emergency room doctors were not willing to withdraw futile life-support systems, owing to the absence of clear regulations in the Natural Death Act.

Under the Natural Death Act Revised Rules, dying and the terminally ill patients who are diagnosed by at least two physicians (one of whom must be a specialist in the disease or condition) may exercise their free will to sign consent forms authorizing withdrawal of cardiopulmonary resuscitation when they become incompetent. Under the revised regulations, the physicians in end-of-life care can withdraw the futile treatment with the patient's consent signed beforehand.

The Revised Rules for the Natural Death Act empower the patient's decision in a more practical way and protect the dignity of the dying. Frontline medical staffs are also in a better position, legally and practically, to deal with the dying patient. Following the revised rules, the most important issues in the next step are how to reinforce the notion of "advance care planning" and "signing the will in advance," and to advocate hospice and palliative care. Public education regarding these issues will be the focal point of missions in the future.

Regulation of Hospice and Palliative Care

In order to establish standards for research on end-of-life care, the Taiwan Academy of Hospice Palliative Medicine set up a monitoring and audit body: the Hospice Joint Ethics Board (HJEB, *An Ling Huan He Yi Liao Lun Li Wei Yuan Hui*). According to its charter, it is to establish policies and regulations for hospice and palliative care research; establish norms for medical ethics for the country; and regulate protection of the rights and interests of patients and families in the research process. In the future, when researchers approach hospice and palliative care units, the units will apply to the HJEB for approval, thus ensuring that the interests of patients are not jeopardized during the research process.

The Taiwan Academy of Hospice Palliative Medicine was appointed by the Department of Health, Taiwan, to execute a Hospice Quality

Assurance Program in 1999. The objectives of this program are to standardize and continue assessments of hospice palliative units, formulating standard guidelines to ensure the quality of hospice palliative care. Furthermore, this assessment is to be used to assist more medical institutions to establish hospice palliative care units. The assessment of hospice inpatient units and home-care programs includes such items as organization structure, continuity of care, clinical management, manpower, qualification of professionals, environment, facility and equipment, teamwork, audits, symptom control, education and training, and communication.

In 2002, 29 inpatient units and 37 home-care programs were assessed. The inpatient units had 2 that were ranked A (best), 11 that were ranked B, 12 that were ranked C, and 4 units that failed (D). Home-care programs had 14 ranked A, 10 ranked B, 10 ranked C, and 3 ranked D (failure). Payments by the Bureau of National Health Insurance are made only for units and programs meeting A through C quality standards. Meanwhile, a series of auditing standards have been validated by the accreditation committee of TAHPM, and executed throughout the country, to supervise and ensure quality standards in hospice palliative care.

In 2000, a formal examination and assessment of physicians as specialists in palliative medicine by the Board of Hospice and Palliative Medicine in Taiwan commenced. The Assessment Regulations for Board Certification of Palliative Medicine (*An Ling Huan He Yi Liao Zhuan Ke Yi Shi Zhen Shen Ban Fa*) provide that physicians who are members of the Taiwan Academy of Hospice Palliative Medicine with a specialty in clinical medicine, and are certified by the Department of Health, are qualified to participate in the specialist assessment program if they have had hospice and palliative medical training—locally or abroad—for at least 3 months and have accumulated at least 200 credits in continuing education programs recognized by TAHPM. Those with overseas specialist certification recognized by TAHPM also qualify. The assessment consists of two parts: a written examination and an oral examination. The scope of assessment embraces key topic areas and methodologies in hospice and palliative care, including cancers and related symptoms; treatment and assessment of terminally ill patients; principles of dealing with the social, psychological, and spiritual disposition of patients; and ethical and legal principles. The Board of Hospice and Palliative Medicine certificate is valid for 6 years, and may be extended for a further 6 years following expiration. Through 2003, 147 physicians passed the examination and were certified as specialists in palliative medicine.

In 2001, the 4th Asia-Pacific Hospice Conference was held in Taipei. The 806 participants included 576 from Taiwan. Other delegates came from the United Kingdom, the United States, Australia, New Zealand, India, Pakistan, Japan, Hong Kong, Singapore, Macau, Malaysia, Korea, Vietnam, Indonesia, and the Philippines. This conference not only promoted the exchange of academic and clinical information, it also increased the visibility of the hospice movement in Taiwan.

Conclusions

Over the past decade, hospice and palliative care, with full government support, has expanded well in Taiwan. This progress includes the development of services, education, and research. However, the relatively large amount of National Health Insurance expenditures for patients in the last year of life in Taiwan still reflects the fact that care for dying patients may have the inappropriate effects of prolonging dying and making death more painful. Hospice and palliative care should be expanded to include all end-of-life cases beyond cancer. The Natural Death Act, makes the options of a living will and a do-not-resuscitate order legal, which can be helpful in reducing unnecessary medical costs, improving the quality of care, and retaining the patient's autonomy at the end of life. In local cultural practice, family-oriented decision making, especially at the end of life, should be emphasized and respected. Good communication among patients, families, and medical professionals can be helpful in achieving the best quality of life for patients and their families.

Acknowledgments

The author thanks Professor Ole Döring for his editorial comments and help with revisions and Ching-Yu Chen, Wen-Yu Hu, Daniel Fu-Chang Tsai, and Dr. Enoch Yueng-Liang Lai for editorial contributions.

References

Chen, C. Y. 1998. "The Expenses of Inpatient Hospital Care for the Elderly at the End of Life in Taiwan" (master's thesis). Taipei: Institute of Public Health, National Yang-Ming University.

Chiu, T. Y. 1997a. "The Attitude toward Terminal Care in Taiwan." In *Annual Report of the National Science Council*, Taipei.

Chiu, T. Y. 1997b. "Pain Control in Terminal Cancer Patients." *Formosan Journal of Medicine* 1: 198–208.

Chiu, T. Y. 2003. "The Strategies to Implement 'Natural Death Act' in Taiwan." *Report of National Science Council*, Taipei.

Chiu, T. Y., and G. Ohi. 1995. "The Attitudes Toward Terminal Care in Rural Communities in Taiwan and Japan: A Comparative Study." University of Tokyo, MA Thesis.

Chiu, T. Y., W. Y. Hu, and C. Y. Chen. 2000a. "Prevalence and Severity of Symptoms in Terminal Cancer Patients: A Study in Taiwan." *Support Care Cancer* 8: 311–313.

Chiu, T. Y., W. Y. Hu, S. Y. Cheng, and C. Y. Chen. 2000b. "Ethical Dilemmas in Palliative Care: A Study in Taiwan." *Journal of Medical Ethics* 26 (5): 353–357.

Chiu, T. Y., W. Y. Hu, B. H. Lue, S. Y. Cheng, and C. Y. Chen. 2001. "Sedation for Refractory Symptoms of Terminal Cancer Patients in Taiwan." *Journal of Pain Symptom Management* 21 (6): 467–472.

Department of Health, The Executive Yuan, Republic of China. 1975. *1974 Vital Statistics, Republic of China*. Taipei: Department of Health.

Department of Health, The Executive Yuan, Republic of China. 1992. *1991 Vital Statistics, Republic of China*. Taipei: Department of Health.

Department of Health. 2002. *Taiwan Public Health Report 2001*. Taipei: Department of Health, p. 7.

Ger, L. P., S. T. Ho, J. J. Wang, and C. H. Cherng. 1998. "The Prevalence and Severity of Cancer Pain: A Study of Newly-Diagnosed Cancer Patients in Taiwan." *Journal of Pain Symptom Management* 15: 285–293.

Ginzberg, E. 1980. "The High Cost of Dying." *Inquiry-Journal of Health Care* 17: 293–295.

Hu, W. Y., T. Y. Chiu, B. H. Lue, C. Y. Chen, C. Y. Hsieh, and Y. C. Chen. 2001. "An Educational Need to 'Natural Death Act' in Taiwan." *Journal of Medical Education* 5 (1): 21–32.

Hu, W. Y., T. Y. Chiu, R. B. Chuang, and C. Y. Chen. 2002. "Solving Family-related Barriers to Truthfulness in Cases of Terminal Cancer in Taiwan: A Professional Perspective." *Cancer Nursing* 25 (6): 486–492.

Lai, Y. L. 2003. "Hospice and Palliative Care in Taiwan," paper presented at the 5th Asian-Pacific Hospice Conference, Japan.

Liu, C. N., and M. C. Yang. 2002. "National Health Insurance Expenditure for Adult Beneficiaries in Taiwan in their Last Year of Life." *Journal of the Formosan Medical Association* 101: 552–559.

Lin, C. C., and S. E. Ward. 1995. "Patient-related Barriers to Cancer Pain Management in Taiwan." *Cancer Nursing* 18: 16–22.

Scitovsky, A. A. 1994. "The High Cost of Dying Revisited." *Milbank Quarterly* 72: 561–591.

Yao, C. A., T. Y. Chiu, W. Y. Hu, R. B. Chuang, S. Y. Cheng, L. T. Lee, and C. Y. Chen. 1997. "A Study of Initial Assessment of Palliative Care: The Viewpoints of Caregivers." *Chinese Journal of Family Medicine* 7: 174–81.

Zweifel, P., S. Felder, and M. Meier. 1999. "Ageing of Population and Health Care Expenditure: A Red Herring?" *Health Economics* 8: 485–96.

11

End-of-Life Decision Making in Turkey

Sahin Aksoy

As discussed in chapter 1, in almost every country, particularly in the developed countries, the aged population is increasing, putting an extra burden on the health care systems and social services. The diseases encountered in old age are often chronic and long term, which necessitates the provision of health care services in an extended and costly manner. This inevitably raises the problem of the distribution of limited sources (Aksoy 1998). Palliative care is an inseparable part of care for chronic and long-term disease, and thus it needs to be discussed in detail. In the palliative care process, both health care professionals and policy makers are faced with many difficult dilemmas. In this chapter, I present the Turkish case and explain the different aspects of end-of-life decision making in Turkey.

Country Context

Turkey is a nation-state with a population of almost 68 million consisting of people from different ethnic backgrounds. It has a young population, with 55 percent under the age of 20 (Republic of Turkey, Prime Ministry State Institute of Statistics 2002). The major faith tradition in Turkey is Islam (95 percent), though there also are small populations of Jews, Christians, and others. Although Turkey is a secular state by its governmental system, because such a great majority of its population are Muslims, religion plays a significant role in ethical reasoning in the public mind, although not at the official level. Turkey is a unique country in its region because it is a Muslim state that is officially committed to adapting a Western life-style and tradition. The reason for mentioning this is that, in the decision-making process, especially at the end of life, it plays a significant role that will be detailed later.

Health Care Context

Health care reform started in Turkey after the mid-1940s (Akdur 2000). In those postwar years Turkey, like many European countries, was a young republic with a smaller (18 million) and aged population. There were diverse health problems in those years to struggle with, including malnutrition, malaria, pneumonia, tuberculosis, smallpox, and other infectious diseases. Furthermore, the infant mortality rate was very high. As a new republic with large territories, the Turkish Republic needed population growth, and as a result abortion was banned in those years (Ozgen 1984).

The health system was restructured in the Turkish Republic in the 1940s and this system is still in use. Under the new structure, there are three levels in health care provision. The first level is health centers, in which general practitioners (GPs), midwives, and nurses give basic health services and preventive care to the public. These institutions have played an important role in the health awareness of the people. The second level of health care services is provided at state hospitals, and the third level at university and specialist hospitals. In the current Turkish health care system, normally the patients follow this chain. That means that a patient is referred to a state hospital by a GP, and to a university hospital by a specialist if necessary. However, this system does not work very well, and many patients go to directly to a university hospital, thus causing a waste of time and resources.

There are primarily five different kinds of health insurance services in Turkey: The Retirement Fund (*Emekli Sandigi*) for civil servants and their families, The Social Insurance Institution (*Sosyal Sigortalar Kurumu*) for laborers and their families, The Social Insurance Institution for Craftsmen, Tradesmen and Other Self-Employed (*Bag-Kur*) for independent businessmen and their families, a Green Card (*Yesil Kart*) for poor people with no social security and their families, and the private health insurance services. In all services except in the Green Card, the person must pay premiums in order to benefit from these services. These premiums are reasonably affordable and worth paying because the coverage is almost unlimited. Individuals are eligible to receive any service with their insurance, including high-grade operations and intensive care services. Eighty-seven percent of the population is covered by one of these insurance services, and 83 percent is covered by health services. The distribution is 19 percent Retirement Fund, 42 percent Social Insurance Institution, 22 percent Social Insurance Institution Craftsman, Tradesman and Other Self-Employed, and 4 percent others (Republic of Turkey, Prime Ministry State Planning Organization 2001).

Priorities in Health Services

Every country has its own priorities in health services. As suggested in chapter 1, although most attention in the West has focused on the elderly as terminal patients, in some countries the major focus might be on younger adult AIDS patients or on children dying from malnutrition or infectious diseases. Another important category, although much smaller in size, consists of critically ill or extremely low birth-weight babies. In each of these categories, the issues might be similar, but the solutions will differ significantly from country to country. Turkey still has problems in providing basic health services and preventive care, and the high infant mortality rate (39 deaths per 1,000 births) compared with other European countries is an indication of this. Despite these problems, many other services have been quite well developed in recent years. Table 11.1

Table 11.1
Changes in health services in Turkey

Year	No. of in-ward patients in health care institutions	No. of beds in health care institutions	No. of beds per 10,000 patients	No. of patients per physician	No. of stay-days in hospital
1980	961,000	85,000	22	1,650	NA
1990	1,895,000	136,638	24	1,115	6.2
2000	2,673,000	172,449	25.8	826	5.5

Source: Ministry of Health (2001).
NA, not available.

provides some figures on changes over the past several decades (Ministry of Health 2001).

These figures indicate that although they are not yet sufficient, the health care services, especially for inpatients, have improved significantly during this period. These improvements are reflected largely in care for elderly patients and palliative care. In palliative care, as in the rest of the health care, the intrinsic aim is to bring about a "medical good." A "medical good" is used as a blanket term to cover medical treatments such as those that lead to the amelioration or sometimes cure of disease processes, the relief of suffering, the prolongation of life, the dressing of wounds or injuries, and so forth. Palliative care also has extrinsic aims. As a result of their professional experience, those involved in palliation may be able to offer a range of advice and discussion based on practical wisdom generated by their own experiences and their experience of health care and life in general (Randall and Downie 1996). In terms of palliative care, Turkey has limitations. As can be seen in table 11.1, the number of beds per 10,000 patients is only 25.8, compared with 51 in the United Kingdom, 67 in Japan, 97 in Germany, and 101 in France (World Bank 1997). This situation prevents doctors from keeping patients for long stays in hospitals. This especially applies to the terminal patients that need palliative care.

According to the "Guideline for Health Care Services" (Ministry of Health 2001), it is the health center's duty to provide services for patients with chronic and terminal diseases at the first level of health care services. The guideline suggests that personnel in health care centers visit these patients regularly, keep their records, refer them to appropriate health care institutions if needed, plan their nursing care at home, provide their medicine, and guide their families. Despite these guidelines, these services are not well provided owing to lack of personnel and equipment as well as general disorganization.

Hospice Services in Terminal Care

It has been argued that palliative care is a synonym for hospice (Cundiff 1992). The hospice approach to the treatment of a terminally ill patient focuses on relieving the physical symptoms and providing psychological and social support for both patient and family. A hospice seeks to optimize the quality of life of the patient's remaining time. It has been suggested in many studies that having hospice facilities in a country is good for the people who use them. However, there are no hospices in Turkey, except some newly established hospice lookalike nursing homes. When we investigate the reason for this, we see that Turkish tradition plays an important role in preventing the establishment and flourishing of hospices. It is worth noting that in Turkey hospice care is only inpatient.

This author recently conducted a survey among 200 volunteers, half of whom were health care professionals (Aksoy 2003). The samples were chosen from different gender and age groups, professional and social backgrounds, and educational levels. The research was conducted in cities in four different geographical regions of Turkey, namely, Ankara (Middle Anatolia), Izmir (West Anatolia), Sanliurfa (South Anatolia), and Erzurum (East Anatolia). The researchers believe that this survey is a representative indicator of the Turkish perspective on this subject.

They found that 47 percent of the general public would not wish to send their relatives to hospices, even if they were available, since they see this as an indication of disrespect to the parents. This attitude may be due to the traditional belief derived from Islam that is so intimate to Turkish culture. It is important for a traditional Turkish family to look after their parents when they are ill or elderly. It is a duty, not a virtue, for children. Today, despite much degeneration of the cultural framework, respect for parents remains unchanged.

To better understand this, it is worth mentioning that family bonds are still very strong in Turkey. In general, all the children, male or female, stay in the same house with their parents until they marry. Their age or profession mostly does not change this. Especially in lower-income families and in villages, the youngest son is expected to stay with his parents after his marriage. Although this has turned out to be an exception these days, still 2 to 3 percent of married couples live with their parents. It is generally perceived as the duty of sons to look after the parents. Therefore it is seen as an offense against the individual to "send" him or her to a hospice in his last days. Some of the negative responses to the survey question, "Would you prefer your close relatives (parents/husband/wife/children) to stay in hospice in their final days if this service were available?" included "No, I think it is my duty to look after them"; No, it is waste of money"; No, it is not right in our tradition"; My relative may be offended"; He/she may think I do not want him/her"; No, it is a sin to leave him there"; No, it is a waiting room for death"; She may not be well treated"; No, I think to send him there is a kind of punishment."

As far as health care professionals are concerned, they are even more reluctant to let their relatives stay in a hospice (Aksoy 2003). More than half of them (55 percent) said that they would not wish their parents to stay in a hospice. Their main reason for this was that they could provide better care for them at home. Although the great majority of university graduates in the general public prefer to have their relatives stay in a hospice, health care professionals (doctors and nurses) do not favor this.

In our survey, we also asked the general public and the health care professionals, "If you know that you are at the terminal stage of an illness, would you prefer to stay in hospital or would you prefer to go home? Why?" While 54 percent of the general public preferred to stay in a hospital, 64 percent of the health care professionals preferred to go home. The main reason for the first group wanting to stay in a hospital was the hope for better care and not to sadden their relatives at home. On the other hand, the health care professionals preferred to go home because they think that not much can be done in hospitals for patients in terminal stages. It is possible to say that Turkish society is an altruistic one in which individuals always consider the needs of close relatives rather than their own needs. Individuals are mostly ready to sacrifice their comfort for others' convenience.

Decisions regarding the place of care should be made in the context of the partnership between patient and professional; caring relatives must be included in the discussion. While the interests of relatives must be considered by the patient, those interests should not undermine the patient's right to be at home. In Turkey, which is a paternalistic society, decisions are generally made, not by patients, but by the next of kin. However, our research indicated that 55 percent of the public would let the patient decide for him or herself.

There are no statistics on proportion of the population that dies in intensive care units (ICUs), hospitals, hospices, or at home in Turkey. However, our survey showed that there is much uncertainty on this matter (Aksoy et al. 2002). While 42 percent of general public think that terminal patients are sent to their homes, 70 percent of the health care professionals responded that they are kept in the hospital. Therefore, it is hard to obtain an accurate proportion, but it is possible to estimate that the majority of terminal patients die in their homes. If they die in hospitals, they are not in intensive care units. K. Akpir, an anesthesiology professor in one of the biggest university hospitals in Turkey, says that "Patients are not admitted to ICUs to let them die under the best of medical care. ICUs are not meant to be agony rooms. In fact patients with no chance of survival should not be admitted to ICUs" (Akpir 2001: 28). As an experienced physician, Akpir says that Turkish society is mystical and emotional. There are two types of patients. One group says "do whatever is needed," which means using all available facilities whether this is beneficial or not. The other group, defined as "accept the destiny," does not participate in the decision making, but rather leaves it to the doctors.

Decision Making at the End of Life

Autonomous patients can choose the extent to which they wish to participate in decisions about treatment; if they wish to be fully involved, they are adequately informed. However, nonautonomous patients are unable to participate in balancing the benefits against burdens and risk in the particular situation. Information from relatives about the patient's wishes, values, and priorities is important in establishing the magnitude and significance of the benefits and harms for the particular patient. Advance directives are suggested as an alternative to this situation. People are encouraged to write advance statements that are followed in terminal care. However, advance statements are difficult to write and might prove difficult to interpret. The patient's wishes should be respected with regard to valid and applicable refusals of treatment, but advance statements cannot bind caregivers to provide treatment that they feel is wrong (Randall and Downie 1996).

There is no legal basis for making binding advance directives in Turkey. It is not even legal to give do-not-resuscitate (DNR) orders. However, this does not mean that this is not practiced in clinics. Many doctors and nurses in anesthesiology and resuscitation departments reported to us that voluntary and involuntary DNR orders are commonly used in ICUs and the wards. Therefore, there is little purpose surmising whether advance statements and DNR orders are legally binding because there is an apparent disparity between what the law allows and the custom and practice among physicians. Although there are no statistical data from Turkey to cite, from our clinical experience and research results, it is clear that not only health care professionals in terminal and critical units but also in other clinics support and practice DNRs. It is obvious that this causes ethical dilemmas and guilt among health care professionals. Therefore it is important to have a national discussion of this issue and make a law on advance directives and DNRs. For this reason, some Turkish bioethicists have suggested the necessity of formalizing advance statements and DNR orders (Oguz 2001). Oguz argues that with a good application of DNR orders, in light of the concept of "futility of treatment," the number of euthanasia requests will decrease.

Euthanasia is another ethical issue related to end-of-life decision making. The first discussions over euthanasia began in Turkey in the 1990s. Official religious authorities and medical associations declared euthanasia unacceptable. In those days, there were very few people who supported euthanasia (Oguz 1996). However, since that time, research conducted in various medical centers has indicated that health care professionals, especially nurses, support both assisted suicide and euthanasia (Bahcecik et al. 1998; Akcil et al. 1998; Ersoy and Altun 2001).

Despite these findings, both passive and active euthanasia remain unlawful under Turkish Criminal Law. While passive euthanasia is considered unintentional killing by law (Turkish Criminal Law, Article 455), active euthanasia is punishable as intentional killing (Turkish Criminal Law, Article 448) (Artuk 2001). As in all divinely revealed religions, euthanasia is absolutely forbidden in Islamic doctrine (Rispler-Chaim 1993). The trend among health care professionals and educated people in supporting active euthanasia can only be interpreted as their falling away from traditional and religious values (Aksoy 2000). As mentioned earlier, with a tendency to be mystical and emotional, and believing in predestination, Turkish people believe that whatever is written in the destiny for this world will be experienced. Therefore, extra efforts at the terminal stage of illnesses may be interpreted as a fight against destiny.

For this reason, the majority of Turkish people are in favor of voluntary passive euthanasia, although not the active form.

One of the major reasons for requesting euthanasia is unbearable pain. Thus the availability of pain management facilities is important in health care institutions. Most of the general public believes that physicians and nurses do all that is humanly possible to control pain from cancer or other fatal diseases. However, few people realize that most physicians should be significantly better trained than they are to treat the physical and psychological symptoms associated with terminal illness. As a result, many people develop a sense of hopelessness, thinking that little can be done to relieve the pain and suffering of the dying process (Cundiff 1992).

In Turkey, pain management services are usually run by anesthesiology departments. However, in recent years, some centers set up new departments dealing exclusively with pain management. Although anesthesiology specialists are competent to relieve pain in terminal illnesses, most medical and nursing schools do not teach palliative care and pain management at the desired level; therefore the general public in Turkey has fears regarding pain associated with cancer and terminal illnesses.

Health Care Costs

Unfortunately, there are no data available for Turkey about the proportion of health care costs expended in last 6 or 3 months of life. Nevertheless, it is not unreasonable to assume that the costs will depend on the nature of the illness and the place of treatment. Our research indicated that Turkish doctors and patients, as well as families, are quite realistic. Cundiff notes that in the United States, "Unfortunately, many patients with advanced cancer are needlessly resuscitated and placed on life support systems when there is no reasonable hope of recovery. This is simply bad medicine" (Cundiff 1992: 12). In terms of that definition, we can say "bad medicine" is not practiced in Turkish hospitals because the patients are not kept for long on life-support systems. Limited resources and the lack of sufficient health care personnel may contribute to this, but the belief in predestination and the desire not to be a burden on others is the main reason for this attitude.

In many countries in the West, dying is increasingly not a natural phase of life, but a time that people spend in social and emotional isolation in a hospital. Although the major part of health care budgets is spent on people in the last year of life, and specifically in the period immediately before death, a growing number of patients are now starting to seek low-technology treatment in order to be able to die with dignity. There is also a widening debate in many countries about the control people have, or should have, over their own death, a question that raises a great many difficult ethical issues (World Health Organization 1999).

We asked the general public and the health care professionals if age should play any role in decision making at the end of life (Aksoy 2003). The responses from both groups were similar: 45 percent of each group said that age should play a role in decision making at the end of life. This result was a bit surprising. We were expecting that far fewer people would say this. We assume that the present economic crisis in the country, and the lack of facilities combined with a high unemployment rate, led people to answer in this way.

Autonomy and Paternalism at the End of Life

In the current understanding of modern bioethics, respect for autonomy of the patient is a primary obligation. Patients want to be in the center of the decision-making process, especially at the end of life. It is argued that all patients have a right to know about their illness and available treatments. The first moral foundation of this "right" is our fundamental belief in the value of truth. Human beings live in communities, and since our ability to sustain a community life depends on honest communication, a high value is placed on truth and honesty in dealing with each other. The second derives from the first and applies to the patient–caregiver relationship. If health care staffs in general are not honest with patients, the fundamental relationship of trust between patients and caregivers is undermined. The third foundation rests on the need for information in order to enable patients to make genuine choices about treatment or nontreatment (Randall and Downie 1996).

Honesty and openness is fundamentally important in decision making at the end of life and in fatal diseases like cancer. Today it is believed that the paternalistic attitudes of health care professionals should change and patients should be fully informed about their conditions. Patients should be told at least as much of the truth about their illness as they wish to know. They do not have an absolute right to remain in ignorance of aspects of their illness that can have a major impact on their family, professional caregivers, or the community. However, our research also indicated a very typical attitude in Turkish society on this matter. We asked two questions (Aksoy 2003). The first one was, "If you have a fatal disease like cancer, and you are in a terminal stage of the disease, would you like to know this, or would you prefer it to be told to one of your close relatives?" The second question was, "If one of your close relatives has a fatal disease like cancer, and he is in a terminal stage of the disease, would you like him to know this, or would you prefer to hide it?" Sixty-one percent of the general public and 89 percent of health care professionals wanted to know their own diagnosis, but 58 percent of the general public and 71 percent of health care professionals preferred to hide the diagnosis from their relatives. These replies were quite interesting and clearly reflected a double standard. The majority of people wanted to know their own diagnosis, but did not want to let others know about the real nature of their disease. Although it seems unjust, the reason behind it is quite innocent. People generally think that they can carry the burden of bad news, but that their relatives may not be able to do so. They just do not want their families to be sad. There are also other studies that support our research (Samur et al. 2001). It is possible to say that it is a characteristic of Turkish people to neglect others' autonomy in the name of being more protective.

The training of health care professionals is important for better health care service. We wondered whether doctors and nurses in Turkey are properly trained to deal with terminal and dying patients (Aksoy, 2003). We asked, "Have you had any courses on how to deal with a dying patient or a patient who is terminally ill?" The result was surprising. We found that while all nurses (100 percent) have had a course on this subject, almost none of the doctors (5 percent) have had a course or lecture on how to deal with a dying patient or a patient who is terminally ill. This result demonstrates that although Turkish doctors are well trained in the scientific and medical aspects of medicine, they are not well informed about the psychological and ethical side of it. We have reported this fact to the relevant authorities, and suggested that they institute some courses for medical students on medical ethics and communication skills.

In this chapter I have tried to provide relevant information on end-of-life decision making in Turkey. This topic is emerging as an important subject in medical ethics in Turkey, as it is in other countries covered in this book. Also, as in other countries, cultural and religious traditions are critical in understanding the debate over end-of-life issues. These factors, along with the relative lack of health resources in Turkey, suggest that as in India and Kenya, dying in Turkey will continue to reflect a more natural process, although the pressures for change discussed here will intensify these issues.

References

Akcil, M., N. Bilgili, S. K. Turkan, M. Yardim, and A. N. Yildiz. 1998. "Universite Son Sinif Ogrencilerinin Otanazi Konusundaki Gorusleri" (Views of Final-Year University Students on Euthanasia). In *Proceedings of 3rd National Bioethics Symposium*, edited by S. Pelin, S. B. Arda, G. Özçelikay, A. Özgür, and F. Senler. Ankara: A. U. Yayinlari, pp. 149–158 (in Turkish).

Akdur, R. 2000. *Turkiye'de Saglik Hizmetleri ve Avrupa Toplulugu Ulkeleri ile Kiyaslanmasi* (Health Care Services in Turkey and Their Comparison with EU Countries). Ankara: A. U. Yayinlari.

Akpir, K. 2001. "Yogun Bakim Hastalarinda Hasta Destegi ve Devami ile Ilgili Kararin Verilmesi" (Decision Making on Patient Support and Maintenance in ICU Patients). *Medikal Etik* 3: 28–34 (in Turkish).

Aksoy, S. 1998. "Saglik Kaynaklarinin Dagitiminda ve Tedavi Kararinin Verilmesinde Kullanilan Kriterlerin Etik Tartismasi" (Ethical Discussion of Criteria Used in the Distribution of Health Care Resources). In *Tıbbi Etik Sempozyumu Bildirileri* (Proceedings of Third National Biethics Symposium) edited by S. Pelin, B. Arda, G. Ozçelikay, A. Özgür, and F. Senler. Ankara: A. U. Yayinlari, pp. 419–424 (in Turkish).

Aksoy, S. 2000. "Can Euthanasia Be Part of a 'Good-doctoring'?" *Eubios Journal of Asian and International Bioethics* 10 (5): 152–154.

Aksoy, S. 2003. "Ethical Considerations on the End of Life Issues in Turkey." In *Asian Bioethics in the 21st Century*, edited·by S. Y. Song, Y. M. Koo and D. R. J. Macer. Christchurch, New Zealand: Eubios Ethics Institute, pp. 79–83.

Artuk, M. E. 2001. "Hukukcu Gozuyle Otanazi" (Euthanasia from a Lawyer's Perspective). In *Medikal Etik*, edited by H. Hatemi and H. Dogan. Istanbul: Yuce, pp. 42–60.

Bahcecik, N., S. E. Alpar, Y. Yildırım, G. Temiz, C. Ozen, and S. Keles. 1998. "Hemsirelerin Otanazi Konusundaki Gorusleri" (Nurses' View on Euthanasia). In *Proceedings of 3rd National Bioethics Symposium*. Edited by S. Pelin, B. Arda, G. Özçelikay, A. Özgür and F. Senler. Ankara: A. U. Yayinlari, pp. 339–348 (in Turkish).

Cundiff, D. 1992. *Euthanasia Is Not the Answer*. Totowa, N.J.: Humana Press.

Ersoy, N., and I. Altun. 2001. "Hemsirelerin Yardimli Intihar Hakkinda Gorusleri ile Ilgili Bir Calisma" (A Study on Nurses' Views on Assisted Suicide). *Turkiye Klinikleri Journal of Medical Ethics* 9: 49–55 (in Turkish).

Ministry of Health. 2001. "Saglik Hizmetlerinin Yurutulmesi Hakkinda Yonerge" (Guideline for Health Care Services). Ankara (in Turkish).

Oguz, Y. 1996. "Euthanasia in Turkey: Cultural and Religious Perspectives." *Eubios Journal of Asian and International Bioethics* 6: 170–171.

Oguz, Y. 2001. "Tip Etigi Acisindan Yasamin Son Doneminde Karar Verme Surecleri" (End-of-life Decision-Making Processes from a Medical Ethics Perspective). *Medikal Etik* 3: 61–67 (in Turkish).

Ozgen, E. 1984. "Cocuk Dusurme ve Dusurtme Suclarinda Ulkemizdeki Son Durum" (The Latest Situation of Abortion in the Country). *Nufusbilim Dergisi* 6: 5–25 (in Turkish).

Randall, F., and R. S. Downie. 1996. *Palliative Care Ethics*. Oxford: Oxford University Press.

Republic of Turkey, Prime Ministry State Institute of Statistics. 2002. http://www.die.gov.tr/ENGLISH/index.html (accessed October 6, 2002).

Republic of Turkey, Prime Ministry State Planning Organization. 2001. http://ekutup.dpt.gov.tr/ekonomi/gosterge/tr/1950-01/ (accessed May 4, 2001).

Rispler-Chaim, V. 1993. *Islamic Medical Ethics in the Twentieth Century*. Leiden, the Netherlands: E. J. Brill, pp. 94–99.

Samur, M., F. C. Senler, H. Akbulut, A. Pamir, and A. Arican. 2001. "Kanser Tanisi Almis Hastalarin Bilgilendirilme Durumu" (The Level of Information on the Patients Who Were Diagnosed with Cancer). In *2nd National Medical Ethics Congress Proceedings*, edited by B. Arda, R. Akdur and E. Aydin. Ankara: A. U. Yayinlari, pp. 510–519 (in Turkish).

World Bank. 1997. *HNP Human Development Network*. Washington, D.C.: World Bank, pp. 44–45.

World Health Organization. 1999. *Health 21*, Copenhagen: World Health Organization, p. 37.

12

Death Policy in the United Kingdom

Richard Ashcroft

The population of the United Kingdom is about 60 million, of whom about 18 percent are over the retirement age, and about 7.5 percent are over 75 years of age. Current projections suggest that by 2020 the total population will rise to about 64 million and the proportion of people over 65 and over 75 will rise to about 19 and 8.7 percent, respectively (Office of National Statistics 2002). These figures suggest that social and medical care of the elderly will grow in importance and that the appropriate medical response to death and dying will become more and more important in policy and politics. In 1999 it was estimated that just over 1 percent of the population dies each year, of whom about 65 percent die in hospitals, 20 percent at home, 8 percent in nursing homes, and 4 percent in hospices (Office of National Statistics 2001).

Palliative Care in the United Kingdom

An important feature of the delivery of palliative care in the United Kingdom is that the greater part of inpatient care is delivered in the private or voluntary sector. Informed commentators note also that the greater part of the financing for palliative care originates in charitable giving (Field and Addington-Hall 1999; Sidell et al. 2000). A large part of palliative care in the primary care or home setting is delivered through charitable-sector organizations, such as the MacMillan nurses, which provide palliative care support in the community in partnership with the National Health Service (NHS), being funded jointly by the state and by charitable giving. Much of this care is free at the point of use, as the NHS itself is. In part this is due to the way palliative care was invented and established in the United Kingdom, which was through the pioneering work in the establishment of charitable and voluntary-sector hospices by Dame Cicely Saunders and others. Saunders, in particular, argued that patients and their relatives ought to develop their own services and raise their own funds as part of validating their role in the dying process (Saunders 1996).

The National Council for Hospice and Specialist Palliative Care Services (NCHSPCS) estimates that palliative care services in the public and voluntary sector currently cost about £300 million (exchange rate fluctuates but in 2004 ~$1.80 US = £1) per year, with about 60 percent (£180 million) of this being funded through the charitable sector. It also notes that most of the capital stock for palliative care facilities (hospices, wards, and care homes) is in the charitable and voluntary sector. NCHSPCS argues that while palliative care services for patients with cancer (and to a lesser extent patients with late-stage AIDS) are reasonably well developed (although stretched), there remains a large population of other patients with serious illness who would benefit from palliative care, but who are unable to receive it for a variety of reasons. Hence there is great inequity of access. NCHSPCS argues that if the NHS were to invest a further £150 million, this inequity could be largely removed, and the dependence of the sector on the vagaries of charitable giving by donation and bequest would be reduced (National Council for Hospice and Specialist Palliative Care 2000). To put this figure into context, the total local and national government expenditure on health services for the United Kingdom in 2000/2001 was £43.87 billion (House of Commons Select Committee on Health 2002). About £21.5 billion of the total NHS budget is spent on hospital care, of which about £15.4 billion is spent on nonday-case admissions to hospital. Of this £15.4 billion, about £1 billion goes to maternity care, £2.6 billion to mental health and learning disability, £0.8 billion to children, £3.6 billion to adults under 65, and £6.8 billion to the elderly.

From these figures, and the data on hospital episodes and hospital activity, it is hard to draw any precise conclusions about the costs of palliative care and intensive care (high-dependence care, critical care), and the NHS does not release cost data broken down this way or the nominal charges used for accounting purposes. Some guesses can be made by examining published data on hospital episode statistics or hospital activity statistics, counting episodes involving referral to specialists in palliative care or in pain management, or specialist beds in palliative care. However, these data may be restricted in various ways (they refer only to NHS data, leaving the private and charity sector out, and they may refer only to England and Wales, leaving Scotland and Northern Ireland out) (Department of Health 2002a, 2001a).

Typically, the figures quoted in the literature are estimates, and generally rather old or ad hoc estimates at that. Nevertheless, it is possible to make some reasonable qualitative judgments about the level of priority given to palliative care in the NHS: It is not regarded as of critical importance. While considerable attention is paid to the diagnosis and therapeutic management of cancer, and considerable press and policy attention is lavished on such issues as error rates in screening programs, relative death rates among countries and among cancers, and so on, the availability of good-quality palliative care either within cancer medicine or outside it is rarely a topic of public debate. Speculating, it is well known to the public and policy makers that palliative medicine exists and it does wonderful work in hospice care and through services such as the MacMillan nurses, and that for a long time Britain led the way in this field. Beyond this "common knowledge" there is little discussion or debate outside the palliative medicine and nursing subprofessions and the charities that provide the bulk of palliative care.

Indeed, it is hard to get a firm grasp on most financial and resource issues in this area. Because almost all health care is provided free at the point of use, only bulk data are available about the relative costs of services within hospitals or at the regional or national level. Hence it is almost impossible to price the cost of a stay in intensive care, for instance, save by crude averaging. The true marginal cost cannot be calculated, mainly because there is no reason to do so since individuals do not pay, and the idea of allocating beds to patients on even quasi-economic grounds is distasteful to almost all patients and professionals in the United Kingdom. Microallocation is done on noneconomic grounds, conceived in terms of "ability to benefit." Sometimes this is reckoned in terms of "added value" using quality-adjusted life years, but this is rarely, if ever, done "at the bedside." More likely it is done at the level of resource allocation among services, decisions at the hospital or national level about purchasing and stocking policies for pharmaceuticals, and so on. The principal instrument of policy seems to be the "bed." In intensive care services, in particular, there are daily debates about how many intensive care beds should be available, when a patient can be admitted to an ICU, and when a patient should be moved out of an ICU in order to free a bed. The location of facilities for high-technology care, and the means of ensuring that patients have access to them, is a matter of intense politics at national and regional levels.

Recently, the U.K. government held a national beds inquiry to examine changes in medicine, demography, and health services and to make projections about the need for beds in hospitals over the next few years (Department of Health 2002b). This inquiry was driven in part by the recognition that beds are expensive and that delayed discharge is a poor use of resources, and in part by findings that other forms of care (such as hospital-at-home schemes; see Grande et al. 1999) are just as effective, somewhat cheaper, and offer reasonable patient and caregiver satisfaction. In light of this policy trend, it may be that the "bed" loses its place as the key indicator of NHS provision and performance, although it is too early to tell. In the short term, Department of Health figures suggest that up to 11 to 13 percent of elderly patients admitted to a hospital in 2000–2001 had their discharge delayed by such factors as hospital-acquired infections, postoperative complications, iatrogenic harm, or hospital-acquired injury, e.g., falling out of bed and breaking a hip (House of Commons Select Committee on Health 2002). Quite apart from the significance of this figure for the 23,235 people so affected, it suggests that long-stay hospital care of the acutely ill will remain important as a target for policy making.

On this basis, I remain to be convinced that "cost of dying" statistics for the United Kingdom can be meaningfully calculated and quoted. A search of the available literature through Medline and the NHS Center for Reviews and Dissemination Economic Evaluation Database has not provided much enlightenment, save to emphasize that the vast majority of such studies are produced in the United States, where the managed care system puts a premium on being able to price each item of care fairly precisely. Nevertheless, figures such as numbers of beds, relative spending on sectors of the population, and spending on disease group-ings (if correlated with death rates, for example) can give useful indica-tions and suggest pathways for future work.

Active Euthanasia and Suicide

In common with almost all jurisdictions, the killing of another person in the United Kingdom is a criminal offense, even at the competent request of that person. Hence active euthanasia is a criminal offense, and according to the strict letter of the law, it is the offense of murder. Mur-der commands a compulsory life sentence in the laws of England and Wales and normally entails a 12-year term of imprisonment before the convicted person is released "on license" (parole).

So much for the theory! In practice, trials of lay people or medical practitioners for murder in cases of suspected euthanasia are very rare for a number of reasons. First of all, in many suspected cases it is hard to establish whether the person died because of the action of the accused party or because of their illness. Because prosecution for a crime is at the discretion of the director of public prosecutions, who must decide whether to bring a prosecution on the basis of whether the evidence available is likely to secure a conviction, an unknown number of cases are never brought to trial for lack of evidence.

Second, most people involved in euthanasia are, reasonably enough, discreet about it, and where there is no reason to suspect foul play, a postmortem is rarely conducted (unless the death took place in a hospi-tal, where a coroner's postmortem is legally required). Death is pro-nounced and certified by a medical practitioner; in most cases this will be a medical practitioner who has had the care of the patient, and thus he or she will record the cause of death according to his or her best judg-ment. Where the practitioner has been involved in euthanasia, he or she is most unlikely to record this as the cause of death. Where the practi-tioner has not been involved in euthanasia, unless the timing of the death or its circumstances are suspicious, again it is unlikely that the doctor would request a postmortem or call the police just to make sure that the patient was not deliberately killed. In several cases where doctors have admitted to euthanasia, investigations have followed up but rarely (if ever) prosecuted them because of the difficulty of establishing the cause of death years after the fact, of identifying which person's euthanasia had been confessed to, or whether deliberate killing or simply appropriate pain control had been practiced in fact.

Third, even where there is prima facie evidence to believe that the patient was deliberately killed, police and prosecutorial practice rarely lead to a charge of murder being pressed. In many of the well-known cases of euthanasia, unless there is reason to think that the killing was in fact nonconsensual or there was an ulterior motive (for instance, financial gain, or escape from an intolerable burden of caring for the patient), for the most part lesser charges that do not attract a mandatory life sentence (or indeed a mandatory custodial sentence of any kind) are normally preferred. For example, people have been prosecuted for manslaughter, attempted murder, assisting suicide, administration of a noxious substance, and other lesser offenses, such as obstructing the course of justice.

Fourth, juries have shown themselves unwilling to convict people they see as "mercy killers." The prosecution, conviction, and sentencing of lay people is sometimes more severe than where the accused is a doctor because doctors are seen as especially trustworthy and empowered to make difficult decisions with special knowledge and experience. Other times these are less severe in lay than in medical cases because the doctor is seen as failing in his or her professional responsibility, or because the layperson's desperation and vulnerability may be transparently obvious (Huxtable 2002). In other words, the application and administration of the law to active euthanasia is very far from being as clear-cut as the letter of the law implies. This failure to apply the law to protect a fundamental human right to life has led many prolife commentators to hint at a liberal conspiracy that is edging us down the slippery slope toward publicly mandated killing. By the same token, it has led proeuthanasia campaigners to protest at the unfairness and arbitrariness of the machinery of law that treats formally similar cases in substantively different ways.

A high-profile recent case of this involved Diane Pretty, a patient suffering from the latter stages of motor neuron disease, who petitioned the courts for a judgment that the Director of Public Prosecutions violated her human right to life (which she interpreted to encompass her right to end her life in a manner of her own choosing) by failing to issue a declaration that her husband would not be prosecuted should he assist her in ending her life. This case eventually was decided by the European Court of Human Rights, which determined that her legal human rights were not violated, and that prosecutorial discretion did rightfully lie in the hands of the Director of Public Prosecutions, notwithstanding the legal permissibility of active voluntary euthanasia in Holland and Belgium. An interesting point is that the Dutch public policy on euthanasia is to permit the exercise of prosecutorial discretion in almost exactly the way requested by Mrs. Pretty. Providing certain guidelines were adhered to, the Dutch public prosecutor would bring no charges after the death of the person whose life had been ended. The significant difference between the Dutch policy and the Pretty case was that one condition the Dutch policy required was that the suicide be physician assisted.

Suicide and Assisted Suicide

Historically, a number of important points can be identified as framing current U.K. euthanasia and suicide policy. Central to most discussion in this area is the Suicide Act of 1961, which decriminalized suicide. Most students of medicine find the idea that suicide could have been a crime quite comical (how could it be prosecuted?). But in unsuccessful attempts at suicide, the offense of attempting suicide could be charged; and in successful cases, the shame and stigma that still attaches in many people's minds to suicide was simply given public expression. Today, great effort is often expended on trying to avoid the verdict of suicide in coroners' courts; and historically suicide, as a sin against God, could be a basis for denying someone a Christian burial.

The removal of criminal stigma from suicide can be understood largely as a reflection of the medicalization of suicide; suicidal ideation being increasingly understood as either a rational response to intolerable circumstances (in particular, to unmanageable mental or physical suffering) or as a frankly irrational wish, best managed through psychiatric care. The first modern Mental Health Act predated the Suicide Act by 2 years (1959), interestingly enough, with provisions for the "sectioning" (compulsory detention under a "section" of the Mental Health Act) of people believed to pose a risk of harm to themselves. (Mental health law provisions for this predate this act, but the context of legal reform here is important.)

The Suicide Act of 1961 removed the criminal stigma from the individual, but redefined and reinforced the offense of aiding, abetting, counseling, or procuring suicide. It applies directly to assisted suicide in cases where the patient is requesting assistance in ending his or her life—for example, asking for a supply of lethal drugs. It would not apply to negligent failure to notice that a patient was likely to attempt suicide, although liability for civil damages or a charge of manslaughter could well apply. The courts have decided that the offense of aiding, abetting, counseling, or procuring suicide should be restricted to cases where one person advises another to commit suicide, makes materials available to him or her, or drives him or her to suicide so that "(a) the accused knew that suicide was contemplated, (b) he or she approved or assented to it, and (c) he or she encouraged the suicide attempt" (Montgomery 1997: 443). Hence the activities of the Voluntary Euthanasia Society and others to publicize the ways in which someone can end his or her life painlessly are lawful, since their activities are not specific to a particular individual that they have reason to be aware of [*A. G. v. Able* (1984), cited in Montgomery 1997: 442–443]. On the other hand, should one of their members aid, abet, counsel, or procure the suicide of a particular patient at that patient's request, that member would be guilty in law of the offense.

Assisting suicide has often been seen as a distinct and straightforward situation where the law could be reformed relatively easily to relieve an unjust burden on both the suffering patient and their "friend" or doctor alike. The straightforwardness of this seems to lie in the autonomous request of the patient to end his or her life, provided a procedural method can be devised to protect patients from rash acts where their decision may be more properly ascribed to incomplete information or to depression—in other words, a decision that mature reflection or better particulars might reverse—and further to protect patients from coercion or misinformation by desperate or malevolent others. However, the English legal position seems to imply (1) the centrality of the "sanctity of life" so that a patient cannot voluntarily alienate their life from themselves, (2) the impossibility of devising a sufficiently watertight procedural protection of the vulnerable from themselves and others, and (3) the special role of the doctor.

Euthanasia, Pain Control, and the Doctrine of Double Effect

The special role of the doctor lies in the well-known asymmetry between a patient's autonomous right to choose among treatments offered, including the right to refuse any or all of them, and the patient's lack of a right to require or demand a particular treatment from a doctor against that doctor's clinical judgment. The doctor is free to refuse to comply with a patient's request (providing that his or her refusal to offer treatment is neither negligent in the light of recognized medical practice nor unjustly discriminatory in the light of the proper use of NHS resources). Hence, a patient's request that a doctor assist his or her suicide, even were this not a criminal offense, could not bind a doctor unless it was accepted clinical practice to do so; more than this, that it was negligent to fail to comply. The courts and Parliament would be very unwilling to allow this possibility to come to pass. If the law was to change, it is almost certain that some sort of "conscientious objection" clause would be contained in the statute, analogous to that included in the Abortion Act of 1967 that allows doctors to refuse to refer a patient for an abortion on conscientious grounds even if the clinical necessity was established in this patient's case. However, the Abortion Act also requires that the doctor refer the patient to another medical practitioner. In sum, then, from a legal point of view, assisted suicide is scarcely to be distinguished from active voluntary euthanasia.

The central case in active voluntary euthanasia was a notorious murder trial, *R v. Adams* (1957), which established the famous "doctrine of double effect" as a principle of English law (rather than simply an argument in Catholic moral theology). Dr. John Bodkin Adams, a general practitioner in a southern seaside town in England, was the beneficiary in the wills of several of his elderly female patients who died. He was accused of murdering several of these patients, for pecuniary gain, by deliberately increasing the dosage of the opiates used to control their pain. A side effect of a large dose of an opiate drug is that the breathing reflex becomes suppressed, leading in effect to the suffocation of the patient, who may be so sedated that he or she neither notices nor is in a position to protest. At the time of Adams's trial, it was believed that adequate pain control in someone in dire pain might lead one to prescribe a dosage that was so large that the unintended consequence of suffocation would follow as well.

Most palliative medicine specialists now argue that in almost all cases, the level of pain suffered by a patient determines the size of dose of opiates required to control the pain *and* the size of the dose required to induce suppression of the breathing reflex. In other words, if a patient is in extreme pain, he or she can tolerate a very high dose of diamorphine that would kill someone in less pain, without undergoing suffocation. However, knowledge of how to "titrate the dose" of diamorphine is not yet widely known, so that an erroneous dose of opiates could still be given with all the right intentions and the genuinely unintended consequence of death. The open question is whether this would be straightforwardly negligent or whether it involves specialist knowledge that not all doctors can be expected to possess. However that may be, at the time of Adams's trial, the theory of titration of the dosage of opiates was not part of common medical knowledge, and it was not invoked at the trial. Dr. Adams was found not guilty, with the judge summarizing the law thus:

If the first purpose of medicine—the restoration of health—could no longer be achieved, there was still much for the doctor to do, and he was entitled to do all that was proper and necessary to relieve pain and suffering even if the measures he took might incidentally shorten life by hours or even longer. [*R v. Adams* (1957), cited in Montgomery 1997: 440].

In other words, motive matters, as does good clinical practice. The almost equally famous case is *R v. Cox* (1992), involving a doctor who deliberately killed a patient who was suffering agonies as a result of arthritis and had repeatedly asked to be helped to die by an injection of potassium chloride. This case underlines the latter point because it was established that potassium chloride, whose principal effect is to stop the heart beating, had no palliative or therapeutic action, but was solely a lethal substance. Hence, whatever Cox's intentions (which were agreed to be good), clinical practice did not warrant this course of action.

The difficulties of constructing a jurisprudence on the doctrine of double effect are manifold, *pace* Keown (2002). Again consider Cox: his subjective intention was to relieve the suffering of his patient, as was Adams's (we must suppose), leading to the death of the patient. Perhaps Adams hoped his patients would not die; perhaps Cox hoped that his would. But as far as their accounts of their intentions are concerned, the objective of both was "relief of the suffering of my patient." Yet the law does not rest with subjective intentions, because it draws a line between Cox and Adams, arguing that Cox's act led so directly to death that his description of his intention was misstated—his true intention can only have been to cause death. Yet, even allowing that, he intended death in order to relieve his patient's suffering.

While it may be that lawyers, judges, and perhaps juries can navigate these twists and turns of argument, it is doubtful that the practitioner can. A likely outcome is that practitioners are led to deception, coverup, and other forms of dishonesty, or to defensive medicine. It is well known that many patients, for their part, resist being prescribed opiates because they fear that the sole purpose of opiates is to kill them, and they distrust the explanations given by doctors. This is not irrational if a practice of incomplete or misleading disclosure or recording in the notes is encouraged by the vicissitudes of legal interpretation and prosecution practice. The hope in all this is that as skills of palliative care and pain control become more widely disseminated in the medical and nursing profession, knowledge of good prescribing practice will obviate the need to appeal to the doctrine of double effect.

So much for active killing of patients at their request! Killing patients who do not want to be killed or who are in no position to say anything because of their incapacity is much more clearly unlawful, as the notorious cases of Dr. Harold Shipman (who is now estimated to have murdered more than 200 of his patients) and of nurse Beverley Allitt (detained at Her Majesty's pleasure in a special hospital for the criminally insane after killing several children in her care as a result of her suffering from Munchausen's syndrome by proxy) remind us. The care of the incompetent and the vulnerable in the NHS causes regular concern, but more for reasons of abuse, neglect, or scarcity of resources than from any suspicion of unlawful killing from motives connected with their health (compare Burleigh 1994, 1997).

Refusing Treatment and Advance Directives

Most public policy in the United Kingdom during the recent decade in this area has been concerned with the withholding or withdrawal of life-sustaining care. The simplest case is the case of advance directives or living wills. A competent patient has a right to refuse any medical treatment, even at the risk of his or her life. This is more complicated in the case of children under 18, who for various reasons, even where they are highly mature, have not been permitted by the courts to refuse lifesaving or life-sustaining medical treatment, but may be permitted to consent to it, even against their parents' wish (British Medical Association 2001). Similar problems arise in cases of the mentally ill or learning disabled (see Montgomery 1997). In essence, the criminal and civil laws protect individuals from being "touched" by another person without their consent, even where the intentions of that other person are honest and honorable, and this includes medical treatment.

As noted in other chapters, an advance directive is a document stating that the person to whom it refers refuses to undergo a certain treatment or range of treatments under specified circumstances. Provided the document is clearly stated, applicable in the circumstances, and was drawn up by the patient while competent and when appropriately informed about his or her options and the consequences of the document, then it counts as validly as a refusal made contemporaneously with the offer of treatment.

There is no statute or case law dealing with the advance directive as such, but in the case of *Re T*, concerning a Jehovah's Witness minor who refused a blood transfusion through an advance directive on religious grounds, the presiding judge stated in an *obiter dictum* (i.e., a collateral opinion) that had T been an adult, then this advance directive would have been binding (*Re T* 1992). It is widely accepted that these advance directives are binding, and although occasionally attempts have been made to put them on a statutory footing, or, alternatively, to create legal proxy decision makers (who can use the so-called "substituted judgment" test), public policy in Parliament and the courts has been to leave it to professional bodies to devise appropriate guidelines.

Advance directives, however, can be problematic. Sometimes they fail to be sufficiently specific, leaving the door open for them to be ignored. Most frequently, doctors in emergency care settings only become aware of them after treatment has begun. There is a powerful theoretical worry that people will compose an advance directive and then it will lie on file long after it ceases to be pertinent to the patient's current medical condition (they may have gotten better, or they may have become reconciled to their condition). Yet, the advantages are generally agreed to outweigh the risks, and many organizations have drafted model advance directives or encourage patients to consider drafting one. The most famous example here is the Terence Higgins Trust, the largest and most well-known charity for people with HIV/AIDS, which popularized advance directives in the 1980s and 1990s. However, because treatments for HIV have become highly effective in halting or slowing its progression, and as a number of hospices for people dying of AIDS have been forced to close or diversify for want of sufficient patients needing their services, advance directives have ceased to be a major part of the trust's activities.

Statistics on advance directives in the United Kingdom are not available, but aside from the relatively small number of people who have a serious neurodegenerative disorder, a terminal illness, or a relative with either of these, or professional experience in dealing with them, advance directives have not become widespread. In practice, this is only to be expected, not only because people do not care to think about such things, but also because the requirement that the advance directive be quite specific makes drawing one up very difficult for persons who are both well and not at appreciable risk of any particular disease.

Withholding Treatment and Do-Not-Resuscitate Orders

The counterpart of the advance-directive is the do-not-resuscitate order. While "DNR" or "No Code" or "Not for 333" or their equivalent has been written on the medical notes of inpatients for many years, the decision was rarely, if ever, discussed with patients. In part this was because a doctor cannot be obliged to offer a treatment that he or she does not think is in that patient's interests. In part, it was also due to the hierarchical nature of medical teams, according to which junior staff are expected to carry out the instructions of their superiors, at least presumptively, and need to know what those instructions are if their superior is not present for some reason or other. Also, the subject was often not raised because it was felt to be upsetting to patients to be told that their health was so fragile that they were not only at risk of heart or lung failure, but also that they might either not survive resuscitation or have such poor health afterward that it was not "worthwhile" to attempt it. This relies on so-called "therapeutic privilege," which permits doctors not to disclose information to their patients if they believe that the information itself might damage that patient's health.

In 2000, there was a public controversy about DNR orders when a 65-year-old female patient in good health who was in the hospital for a relatively minor operation discovered on discharge that DNR had been written into her notes. Her case was taken up by Age Concern England, a large charity-cum-pressure group for the elderly, which discovered numerous similar cases (Ebrahim 2000). Many commentators have pointed out that the success rate for cardiopulmonary resuscitation is low, the procedure is undignified, and it medicalizes death (Timmermans 1999). However, be that as it may, there was no case for a purely age-related decision, unconnected to prognosis or baseline health. Age Concern England very reasonably pressed for a reform of the practice of DNR decisions, and linked this to evidence they had collected about abuse of elders in hospital and denial of services to people on irrelevant age-related criteria (Age Concern England 2000).

In response, the Department of Health issued guidance on DNR orders, requiring them to be discussed by a senior member of the admitting medical or surgical team when any patient was admitted to a hospital. This has provoked great unhappiness in the medical profession, which argues that this may lead to absurd conclusions. The level of compliance with the guidance has not been audited, but I suspect it is not good. Nevertheless, this policy applies both to the NHS and to independent institutions (Department of Health 2000, 2002c).

Withholding Treatment and Discrimination Against the Elderly

The debate has been taken up in the wider context of the government's National Service Framework for Older People, an overall policy for health and social care for older people that sets quality standards and targets with the aim of reducing discrimination against older people (Department of Health 2001b). However, the focus is on ending abuse and "attitudinal" problems concerning older people. The evidence base for strictly age-related denial of services to older people is negligible, although some exists, and most people believe that it occurs more or less systematically (see Bowling et al. 2001). This form of discrimination is notoriously difficult to document or prove, especially when trying to disentangle denial of services based on poor prognosis from denial of services based on chronological age. For the most part we depend on inferences either from patients' or families' reports of their own experience (as with Age Concern England 2000), or surveys of attitudes to hypothetical cases (for example, Neuberger et al. 1998). And some people hold that age-related discrimination is not in any case unjust; for example, see Williams (1997) and for the contrary view see Harris (1987) and Evans (1997). It is telling that the literature on the prevalence of age-related denial of service or discrimination tends to turn back very quickly to Aaron and Schwartz's (1984) comparison of allocation practices in the United Kingdom and the United States, where the evidence presented refers to age-based treatment cutoffs that were then explicit and now are nowhere expressly stated. In sum, we are in the dark, and 20-year-old evidence provides no illumination.

Withholding Treatment as Rationing

According to most accounts, it is a mistake to link the debate on rationing to the debate on "passive euthanasia" (i.e., euthanasia by nontreatment or inaction). However, in the public's mind, and in the arguments of "prolife" antieuthanasia campaigners, these debates are linked. On a "macro" level, the public is inclined to see denial of service as a betrayal of the trust they vest in the NHS—as a particularly gross form of neglect. However, older people are frequently reported to be relatively self-denying in terms of aggressive treatment (Williams 1997; Kennelly and Bowling 2001). So what seems to matter is the locus of decision making and trust, rather than the content of the decision making per se.

Historically, passive nonvoluntary euthanasia by neglect has on occasions been a precursor to active involuntary euthanasia (i.e., neglect of the incompetent leading to murder of the competent and nonconsulted) (Burleigh 1994). The antieuthanasia campaigners are always alert to the risk of collapsing the category of "poor in quality of life" into the category of "life unworthy of life." In caring for individual patients, it is frequently difficult to reassure them that a DNR order or a judgment that a treatment will not be beneficial—and, most of all, that a decision to withdraw nutrition or hydration—are not grounded in "rationing," or in "giving up on the patient," but rather are grounded in their lack of efficacy for a particular patient at a particular time. More generally, analytical difficulties in defining "clinical effectiveness" as a criterion for deciding which treatments can be offered by the NHS, and to which categories of patient, challenge the very idea of individualized care. It is certainly the case that ineffective or unsafe treatments should be eliminated, but defining the scope and cutoff for "effectiveness" criteria is an operational necessity for doctors, the NHS, and the National Institute of Clinical Excellence, which is charged with making this kind of technology assessment (Ashcroft 2002).

For this reason, stringent efforts have been made by the courts and by the government and professions to ensure that guidance for the withdrawal and withholding of treatment is based strictly on the need (i.e., capacity to benefit) of the individual patient. Two classic examples of this illustrate the main points. The case of Child B (Jaymee Bowen) commanded considerable attention in the press because it concerned a young girl dying of leukemia, that had proved refractory to treatment. After the Cambridgeshire Health Authority refused to pay for a last-chance experimental therapy, her father tried to get the courts to force the Health Authority to pay. This the court refused to do, partly on the grounds that it was the Health Authority's responsibility to manage its own resources responsibly. It was not a public law matter unless they could be shown not to be deciding reasonably and responsibly. But the main reason for the court's refusal was that this experimental therapy had a very low prospect of success and would impose additional burdens on the child, and hence that it was not in the child's interest to receive the treatment [*R v. Cambridge DHA, ex p. B* (1995), cited in Montgomery 1997: 64–65]. The important points here are (1) the deference to clinical judgment about what was in the child's best interest (although this was tested in evidence, it was still determinative in the last instance) and (2) the use of public law standards for determining whether this was in the court's jurisdiction. The court could overturn a manifestly discriminatory policy, but would not intervene in the reasonable use of appropriately assigned discretionary powers.

Another classic case is the case of Tony Bland. Bland was a victim in a major football stadium disaster, in which he suffered brain damage and went into a coma that led to a persistent vegetative state (PVS). His parents (and doctors) believed that he would never regain consciousness and was to all intents and purposes no longer a person, although his physical body continued to function. Eventually, the House of Lords (the highest court in the United Kingdom) determined in a 3 to 2 opinion that his life support could be switched off and nutrition and hydration stopped. Bland eventually died, without apparent suffering or regaining mental function [*Airedale NHS Trust v. Bland* (1993), Montgomery 1997: 50–53, Jennett 2002]. In this case, it was eventually determined that Bland could not be said to have any interests at all because his capacity for consciousness had been destroyed. The law lords also decided that this was not euthanasia because no action leading directly to death was involved (invoking the acts and omissions distinction). The most controversial points were the robustness of the diagnosis of PVS and the proposition that *artificial* nutrition and hydration were medical treatments rather than basic care.

Although the Human Rights Act was not then in force, the United Kingdom, as signatories to the relevant European Convention, nonetheless followed the practice of taking it into account in major court decisions. Since the passage of the Human Rights Act of 2000, the applicability of its provisions to people in PVS has been tested, and the Bland decision remains the relevant precedent in law. In light of this, the British Medical Association (the doctors' professional association) and the General Medical Council (the medical profession's statutory

regulatory body) have issued guidance setting out the legal and professional requirements to be met by doctors considering withdrawing or
withholding life-sustaining treatment or nutrition and hydration. It remains the case that PVS patient cases must be heard by the courts where
their interests are represented by the official solicitor, a public law officer
whose brief is to represent people who are legally incapable of repre-
senting themselves because of incompetence or incapacity (Montgomery
1997; Jennett 2002; British Medical Association 2000; General Medical
Council 2002).

Conclusions

The long road through the maze of U.K. policy on medical death and
dying ends here. There is obviously more that could be said, for instance
on brain death and transplantation policy, or on public health approaches to the prevention of preventable death as a focus of a wider,
informal "death policy" (Price 2000; Lee and Morgan 1994). Decision
making in this area rests with three main parties: the patient him or herself (but not relatives who have no legal authority to consent on the
adult's behalf, no matter how incapacitated he or she may be); the doctor
in charge of the patient's care (and behind the doctor, the doctor's professional bodies that write the guidelines the doctor will follow); and the
courts (and behind them, the common law). Statute law and official
government policy have a relatively small part to play.

The role of the government in shaping the landscape of death and
dying in the United Kingdom is arguably rather small, save in one
respect—costs. Because the government has a large say in directing
financial flows, the death-related consequences of those directions have
to be considered carefully. It remains the case that as far as the attempt
to change service priority is concerned, the essentially pluralist nature
of British medical policy must be taken seriously. As in 1948 when the
National Health Service was established, so today, in the long run the
government can only make decisions that carry the professions with
them (Foot 1999; Webster 2002; Klein 2000).

The power held by patients remains weak, save in some exceptional
areas (witness the radical changes to pathology practice following the

Bristol Royal Infirmary and Royal Liverpool Children's Hospital inquiries (Bristol Royal Infirmary Inquiry 2000; Royal Liverpool Children's Inquiry 2001; Richardson 2001). These two public inquiries involved wholly or in part scandals over postmortem retention of tissue or organs from children, which prompted widespread public outcry. This outcry, the public inquiries, and a relatively populist government together combined to change pathologists' practice, and to extend even further the consent paradigm into health service practice (Department of Health 2002d). How far this extension will continue remains to be seen (O'Neill 2002a,b).

References

Aaron, H. T., and W. B. Schwartz. 1984. *The Painful Prescription: Rationing Hospital Care.* Washington, D.C.: Brookings Institution.

A. G. v. Able. 1984. *All England Law Reports* 1: 277 ff. ([1984] 1 All ER 277).

Age Concern England. 2000. *Turning Your Back on Us. Older People and the NHS.* London: Age Concern England.

Airedale NHS Trust v. Bland. 1993. *All England Law Reports* 1: 821 ([1993] 1 All ER 821).

Ashcroft, R. E. 2002. "What Is Clinical Effectiveness?" *Studies in History and Philosophy of Biological and Biomedical Sciences* 33C: 219–233.

Bowling, A., M. Bond, D. McKee, M. McClay, A. P. Banning, N. Dudley, A. Elder, A. Martin, and I. Blackman. 2001. "Equity in Access to Exercise Tolerance Testing Coronary Angiography, and Coronary Artery Bypass Grafting by Age, Sex, and Clinical Indications." *Heart* 85: 680–686.

Bristol Royal Infirmary Inquiry. 2000. *The Inquiry into the Management of Care of Children Receiving Complex Heart Surgery at The Bristol Royal Infirmary. Interim Report: Removal and Retention of Human Material.* London: The Stationery Office. http://www.bristol-inquiry.org.uk/interim_report/index.htm (accessed August 15, 2002).

British Medical Association. 2001. *Withdrawing and Withholding Life-Prolonging Medical Treatment: Guidance for Decision-Making.* 2nd ed. London: British Medical Association.

Burleigh, M. 1994. *Death and Deliverance: Euthanasia in Germany 1900–1945.* London: Pan.

Burleigh, M. 1997. *Ethics and Extermination: Reflections on Nazi Genocide.* Cambridge: Cambridge University Press.

Department of Health. 2000. *Resuscitation Policy Health Service Circular HSC 2000/028*. London: Department of Health.

Department of Health. 2001a. Hospital Activity Statistics, England: Financial Year 2000–2001. http://www.doh.gov.uk/hospitalactivity/ (accessed August 14, 2002).

Department of Health. 2001b. National Service Framework for Older People London: Department of Health. http://www.doh.gov.uk/nsf/olderpeople.htm (accessed August 14, 2002).

Department of Health. 2002a. *Hospital Episode Statistics, England: Financial Year 2000–2001*. London: Department of Health.

Department of Health. 2002b. *Shaping the Future NHS: Long-Term Planning for Hospitals and Related Services. Consultation Document on the Findings of the National Beds Inquiry: Supporting Analysis*. London: Department of Health.

Department of Health. 2002c. *Independent Health Care: National Minimum Standards Regulations*. London: Department of Health.

Department of Health. 2002d. *Human Bodies, Human Choices: The Law on Human Organs and Tissues in England and Wales—A Consultation Report*. London: Department of Health.

Dickenson, D. L., M. Johnson, and J. Katz, eds. 2000. *Death, Dying and Bereavement*. London: Sage.

Ebrahim, S. 2000. "Do Not Resuscitate Decisions: Flogging a Dead Horse or a Dignified Death?" *British Medical Journal* 320: 1155–1156.

Evans, J. G. 1997. "The Rationing Debate: Rationing Health Care by Age: The Case Against." *British Medical Journal* 314: 822–825.

Field, D., and J. Addington-Hall. 1999. "Extending Palliative Care to All?" *Social Science and Medicine* 48: 1271–1280.

Foot, M. 1999. *Aneurin Bevan: 1897–1960*. London: Orion.

General Medical Council. 2002. Withholding and Withdrawing Life-Prolonging Treatments. London: General Medical Council. http://www.gmc-uk.org/standards/whwd.htm (accessed August 15, 2002).

Grande, G. E., C. J. Todd, S. I. G. Barclay, and M. C. Farquhar. 1999. "Does Hospital at Home for Palliative Care Facilitate Death at Home? Randomised Controlled Trial." *British Journal of Medicine* 319: 1472–1475.

Harris, J. 1987. "QALYfying the Value of Life." *Journal of Medical Ethics* 13: 117–1723.

House of Commons Select Committee on Health. 2002. Public Expenditure on Health and Personal Social Services 2001. Memorandum Received from the Department of Health containing Replies to a Written Question from the Committee HC 242. Tables 2.1.1.1(b), 4.14.10. http://www.parliament.the-stationery-office.co.uk/pa/cm200102/cmselect/cmhealth/242/242m01.htm (accessed August 14, 2002).

Huxtable, R. 2002. "The Rationality, Legality and Morality of Assisted Death," unpublished Ph.D. dissertation, University of Bristol, Bristol, U.K.

Jennett, B. 2002. *The Vegetative State: Medical Facts, Ethical and Legal Dilemmas.* Cambridge: Cambridge University Press.

Kennelly, C., and A. Bowling. 2001. "Suffering in Deference: A Focus Group Study of Older Patients' Preferences for Treatment and Perceptions of Risk." *Quality and Safety in Health Care* 10: 23–28.

Keown, J. 2002. *Euthanasia, Ethics and Public Policy: An Argument against Legislation.* Cambridge: Cambridge University Press.

Klein, R. 2000. *The New Politics of the NHS.* 5th ed. London: Prentice Hall.

Lee, R., and D. Morgan (eds.) 1994. *Death Rites: Law and Ethics at the End of Life.* London: Routledge.

Montgomery, J. 1997. *Health Care Law.* Oxford: Oxford University Press.

National Council for Hospice and Specialist Palliative Care Services. 2000. Draft National Plan and Strategic Framework for Palliative Care: 2000–2005. http://www.hospice-spc-council.org.uk/ (accessed August 8, 2002).

Neuberger, J., D. Adams, P. MacMaster, A. Maidment, and M. Speed. 1998. "Assessing Priorities for Allocation of Donor Liver Grafts: Survey of Public and Clinicians." *British Medical Journal* 317: 172–175.

Office of National Statistics. 2001. *Mortality Statistics: General. Review of the Registrar General on Deaths in England and Wales, 1999.* London: The Stationery Office.

Office of National Statistics. 2002. *Population Trends.* London: Office of National Statistics.

O'Neill, O. 2002a. *Autonomy and Trust in Bioethics.* Cambridge: Cambridge University Press.

O'Neill, O. 2002b. *A Question of Trust: BBC Reith Lectures 2002.* Cambridge: Cambridge University Press.

Price, D. 2000. *Legal and Ethical Aspects of Organ Transplantation.* Cambridge: Cambridge University Press.

R v. Adams. 1957. *Criminal Law Review:* 357 ([1957] Crim LR 357).

R v. Cambridge DHA, ex p. B. 1995. *All England Law Reports* 2: 129 (see both [1995] 2 All ER 129 (CA) and [1995] 1 FLR 1055).

R v. Cox. 1992. *Blackwells Medical Law Review* 12:38 ([1992] 12 BMLR 38).

Re T. 1992. *All England Law Reports* 4: 649, 661 668 ([1992] 4 All ER 649, 661, 668).

Richardson, R. 2001. *Death, Dissection and the Destitute.* London: Phoenix.

Royal Liverpool Children's Inquiry. 2001. *Report.* London: The Stationery Office. http://www.rlcinquiry.org.uk/index.htm (accessed August 15, 2002).

Saunders, C. 1996. *Hospice Mortality* 1: 317–322.

Sidell, M., J. S. Katz, and C. Komaromy. 2000. "The Case for Palliative Care in Residential and Nursing Homes." In D. L. Dickenson, M. Johnson, and J. Katz eds., *Death, Dying and Bereavement.* London: Sage, pp. 107–121.

Timmermans, S. 1999. *Sudden Death and the Myth of CPR.* Philadelphia, Pa.: Temple University Press.

Webster, C. 2002. *The National Health Service: A Political History.* 2nd ed. Oxford: Oxford University Press.

Williams, A. 1997. "The Rationing Debate: Rationing Health Care by Age: The Case For." *British Medical Journal* 314: 820–822.

13

Death and Dying: The American Experience

Janna C. Merrick

Many factors affect how we die and where we die. In the United States, most people die in hospitals, and most are elderly. This chapter begins with an analysis of how terminal care is affected by the absence of a universal health care system. It analyzes how and where Americans die and at what cost. It then turns to a discussion of public policy as it relates to death. Specifically, it traces events in the public debate about terminal care and physician-assisted suicide and analyzes major state and national laws and court decisions of the past 35 years.

Access to Health Care

Unlike most industrialized nations, the United States has no universal health care system. Delivery of health care is deeply entrenched in the private enterprise system, and expenses are paid through third-party payer systems for those having health insurance.[1] In the year 2000, approximately 14 percent of the population, about 38.7 million persons, had no insurance coverage whatsoever (Mills 2001). Even for those who have coverage, many costs are not reimbursed and must be paid by the patient. Most insurance plans, whether private or government sponsored, are "managed care" plans driven by cost containment, with strict limitations on eligible procedures, use of specialists, time allowed for hospitalization, and so forth. Patients' expenses in the United States in 2000 were $707 per capita compared with only $171 per capita[2] in the United Kingdom (G. Anderson et al. 2002).

Despite the difficulties with insurance coverage and access to health care, the World Health Organization reports a life expectancy in the year

2001 of 74.3 years for males and 79.5 years for females. Moreover, child mortality rates[3] were low at 9 deaths per 1,000 live births for males and 7 for females. These rates are comparable to those in other industrialized countries (World Health Organization 2002), but costs are much higher both as a percentage of gross domestic product (GDP) and in actual dollars. For example, in 2000, the United States spent 13 percent of its GDP on health care, while the United Kingdom spent only 7.3 percent (G. Anderson et al. 2002). In actual dollars, the United States spent $4,631 per capita, compared with only $1,763 in the United Kingdom despite almost identical life expectancies and infant mortality rates (G. Anderson et al. 2002).[4]

Causes, Location, and Costs of Dying

In 2003, the Institute of Medicine of the National Academy of Sciences estimated that 2.4 million Americans die annually. The institute argues that as a nation, we "know relatively little about the quality, appropriateness, or costs of the care they receive, or the burden on caregivers and survivors" (Institute of Medicine 2003: 1). With these limitations in mind, this section addresses the causes, location, and costs of death in the United States.

The ten leading causes of death in order of rank are heart disease, cancer (especially lung cancer), stroke, chronic lower respiratory diseases, accidents (especially automobile accidents), diabetes mellitus, influenza or pneumonia, Alzheimer's disease, kidney disease, and septicemia (blood poisoning). Together these diseases account for 80 percent of all deaths (R. Anderson 2001). The causes of death, of course, vary by demographic characteristic, with age being a major variable. For infants less than 1 year, the three leading causes are congenital malformations (including chromosomal abnormalities) premature delivery and low birth weight, and sudden infant death syndrome (SIDS). For persons aged 1 to 34 years, the leading cause of death is accidents. Other leading causes include homicide, suicide, and human immunodeficiency virus (HIV), and cancer. For older Americans, deaths from chronic diseases are more common, with cancer and heart disease as the two leading causes (R. Anderson 2001).

Most terminally ill patients express a desire to die at home, but relatively few actually die there. Pritchard's study of terminally ill patients at five teaching hospitals showed that 56 percent of patients died in acute care hospitals, 25 percent died at home, 9 percent died in nursing homes, 9 percent died in hospices, and 1 percent died en route to the hospital. However, when geographic location is considered, the rates of in-hospital deaths vary from 29 to 66 percent. Among Medicare[5] patients, 39 percent died in hospitals, but again there were variations based on geographic region (Pritchard et al. 1998). A stated preference for dying at home was not a factor in determining where patients died, nor were advance directives (Pritchard et al. 1998). Rather, dying in hospitals was positively correlated with the availability and use of health services in the region, especially the availability of acute hospital care. More Medicare patients die in hospitals in regions with greater numbers of hospital beds. This is moderated by the availability of hospice or skilled nursing care, which reduces the number of in-hospital deaths (Pritchard et al. 1998).

Hospice care may be provided in either a hospice facility or the home. The latter is the most common in the United States. The care is primarily palliative, not curative. Hospice care is covered by Medicare, and in most states, Medicaid.[6] Many private insurers also provide hospice coverage. Hospice care is much more cost-efficient than hospitalization or admission to a skilled nursing facility. The Hospice Association of America reports that in 1997, the costs of home hospice care were approximately $108 per day, compared with hospitalization at $2,121 per day and skilled nursing facility care at $454 per day (Hospice Assn. of America 2003).

National data on hospice use in the United States are unavailable; however, a study of hospice use by Medicare patients is illustrative of its relatively low use. The study reports that 15.5 percent of Medicare patients died in hospices in 1996. The use of hospices varied with a number of demographic factors, including age, race, gender, income, and geographic location. "Younger" persons (aged 65 to 74) were more likely to use a hospice than "older" persons (aged 75 and above), non-blacks more likely than blacks, women were slightly more likely than men, persons with higher incomes more likely than persons with lower incomes, and persons living in urban areas more likely than those living in rural areas. Health care "market" factors also played a role. Hospice use was higher in communities having high managed care penetration, which is probably due to the perception that hospice care is less expensive than hospital care. Hospice use was lower in communities with more hospital beds per capita and higher rates of in-hospital deaths (Virnig et al. 2000).

Hospice use is also affected by physicians' practice characteristics and knowledge of hospice care. Overall, the physicians studied referred about 55 percent of their terminally ill patients for hospice care. Referral varied by specialty, with oncologists referring the largest proportion of their patients (Bradley et al. 2000). This is to be expected since other studies have shown that the overwhelming majority of hospice users have a diagnosis of cancer (Cristakis and Escarce 1996; Hogan et al. 2001). The most common reasons reported for nonreferral were patient or family refusal and/or lack of interest, or a belief by the physician that a hospice was not appropriate (Bradley et al. 2000). Hospice use is on the rise, as evidenced by a significant increase in the percentage of Medicare patients who died in hospices between 1994 (11 percent) and 1998 (19 percent). More than half of Medicare cancer deaths occurred in hospices (Hogan et al. 2001).

There has been much discussion in the United States about the high costs of dying. While there is no national database for the population as a whole, there are good records on Medicare patient costs, and since Medicare patients constitute 80 percent of annual deaths, their records are often used to calculate the costs of dying. A number of patterns are evident. Expenditures for Medicare patients during their last year of life account for approximately one-quarter of Medicare's total outlays (Hogan et al. 2001). This pattern has been fairly stable for nearly 30 years. Moreover, expenditures are five times higher for patients during the last year of life than for patients who do not die during the year (Levinsky et al. 2001), and 40 percent of the last-year-of-life expenditures are incurred during the last month of life ("Costs" 1999). Part of the explanation for this is that persons who die tend to have more diseases than persons who survive. Even when controlled for age and diagnoses, however, those who die have higher costs than those who survive.

Also, end-of-life costs are higher for minorities and for persons living in areas with high rates of poverty. For example, the average per capita last-year-of-life Medicare outlay for 1993–1998 was $25,000 for Caucasians and $32,000 for minorities (Hogan et al. 2001).

Another interesting pattern is that costs for the last year of life decrease as the patient ages, owing to less aggressive treatment, including less frequent hospitalization; fewer admissions to intensive care units; and markedly decreasing use of cardiac catheterization, dialysis, ventilators, and pulmonary artery monitors. Expenditures are highest for those who die in hospitals, followed by those who die in nursing homes. The costs are lowest for patients who die at home. As would be expected, as expenditures for hospitalization decline with age, expenditures for both skilled nursing care and for home health services increase. These patterns are consistent regardless of race, sex, type of care facility, degree of comorbidity and its cause, or place of death (Levinsky et al. 2001). These findings counter the popular belief discussed later that patients are subjected to aggressive but futile treatments that simply prolong the process of dying. To further illuminate this issue, we discuss pain management and palliative care.

Pain Management and Palliative Care

In recent years there has been much discussion of palliative care and the need for improvement[7] in the United States. One area involves the level and quality of pain management. Forty-three percent of Americans will enter a nursing home prior to death, and more than 1.5 million are currently cared for in nursing homes. According to Teno et al. (2001), nearly 15 percent of these patients are in persistent pain at the time of initial assessment, and of these, approximately 41 percent are in severe pain 60 to 180 days later. Thus pain management continues to be a major concern.

In addition to questions of palliative care in nursing homes, there are serious questions about palliative care in hospital settings, as evidenced in research by Cassel and colleagues (2000). These authors searched for the causes of what they describe as the "underdeveloped and undervalued status" of palliative care in hospital settings. While they found some nonfinancial causes, such as Americans' reluctance to deal with death, most causes were related to lack of revenue to pay for palliative care in hospital settings. Specifically, they point to Medicare payment provisions that encourage hospitals to discharge dying patients quickly. This creates a predicament both for hospitals and physicians. Moreover, life-prolonging attempts have better reimbursement, which some may argue leads to more aggressive treatment in futile situations (Cassel et al. 2000).

Dying in the United States: Early Development of Law and Public Policy

For most of American history, discussions about death and dying were taboo.[8] Neither policy makers nor patients and their families openly discussed the circumstances under which patients would die; thus few public policies existed. This scenario began to change in the late 1960s with the publication of On Death and Dying by psychiatrist Elisabeth Kubler-Ross (1969). Her work—which focused on how terminally ill patients were often shunned and lied to about their prognosis for survival—became a triggering event for a public discussion about the roles and needs of terminally ill patients, their loved ones, and their health care providers. Five years later, the first hospice in the United States, initially funded by the National Cancer Institute of the National Institutes of Health, began providing home hospice care in Branford, Connecticut.

In 1975, the case of Karen Ann Quinlan became a major agenda-setting event in Americans' discussion about terminal care. The 21-year-old New Jersey girl lapsed into a chronic persistent vegetative state (PVS)[9] after losing consciousness. She was not brain dead and was placed on a respirator; however, her condition continued to deteriorate. Her family, devout Catholics, attempted to have the respirator removed, but the hospital refused. Her family then initiated litigation seeking termination of life support and appointment of Karen's father as her legal guardian with decision-making power regarding her care.

The effort to disconnect the respirator was opposed by her doctors, the hospital, the county prosecutor, the State of New Jersey, and her guardian ad litem (for the suit). A media frenzy resulted when this opposition became public. The trial court refused the request for withdrawal of

treatment and appointed a stranger as Karen's guardian for medical decision making. Her family appealed the trial court's decision to the New
Jersey Supreme Court, which found that Karen was grossly incompetent
to make decisions about her medical care. However, the court could not
discern what her pre-illness views would have been regarding the withdrawal of life support. Therefore, it found that the best way to protect
her rights was to permit her family members to render their best judgment about what Karen would choose if she were competent (*In the
Matter of Karen Quinlan. An Alleged Incompetent* 70 N.J. 10 [1976]).
Her father was appointed as her guardian and the stranger guardian was
dismissed.

The court then turned to the question of Karen's constitutional rights
to privacy and concluded

that no external compelling interest of the State could compel Karen to endure
the unendurable, only to vegetate a few measurable months with no realistic
possibility of returning to any semblance of cognitive or sapient life.... [T]he
individual's right to privacy grows as the degree of bodily invasion increases and
the prognosis dims. Ultimately there comes a point at which the individual's
rights overcome the State interest (*In the Matter of Karen Quinlan*, 40).

After resolving the issue of Karen's right to privacy, the court turned
to the issue of whether her father, as guardian, could withdraw life support. Noting the paucity of legislative and judicial guidance on this issue,
the court made important distinctions between curative and palliative
care.

We glean from the record here that physicians distinguish between curing the ill
and comforting and easing the dying.... For those possibly curable, [artificial
life-sustaining devices] are of great value, and, as ordinary medical procedures,
are essential.... But in light of the situation in the present case (while the record
here is somewhat hazy in distinguishing between "ordinary" and "extraordinary" measures), one would have to think that the use of the same respirator
or like support could be considered "ordinary" in the context of the possibly
curable patient but "extraordinary" in the context of the forced sustaining by
cardio-respiratory processes of an irreversibly doomed patient (*In the Matter of
Karen Quinlan*, 56).

The court then ordered that life support could be withdrawn if responsible attending physicians believed there was no reasonable possibility of Karen ever emerging from her comatose condition, and the
family agreed to the withdrawal. Prior to discontinuing life support, the

ethics committee of the hospital was to be consulted. Karen was subsequently detached from the life-support system, but despite the prognosis for a quick death, she began to breathe on her own and remained in a persistent vegetative state until her death on June 11, 1985, a decade after lapsing into PVS and 9 years after being detached from the respirator. The tragic case of Karen Ann Quinlan became the turning point in America's public discussion about terminal care, particularly for patients whose conditions were hopeless.

Events continued to fuel this public discussion about America's death policy. In 1983, the President's Commission for the Study of Ethical Problems in Medicine and Biomedical and Behavioral Research published its report entitled *Deciding to Forego Life-Sustaining Treatment.* Its central conclusion was that decisions regarding health care, including the refusal or withdrawal of life-sustaining treatment, rest ultimately with the competent patient exercised through procedures for informed consent.[10] When a patient is no longer competent, a surrogate decision maker—usually a family member—should make the decision that the patient would have made if competent. If there is no evidence of what the patient would want, then the surrogate should make the decision that is in the patient's best interest (President's Commission, 1983).

In 1985, well-known television news correspondent Betty Rollin publicly admitted to assisting in her mother's suicide. Written in powerful and poignant language, *Last Wish* described her mother's battle with ovarian cancer. Rollin writes:

[t]wo hours before my mother killed herself, I noticed she had put on makeup. This shocked me, but it shouldn't have. Whatever the occasion, my mother liked to look her best. That was her way. Just as it was her way to die as she did—not when death summoned her, but when she summoned death (Rollin 1985: 5).

The following year, the debate about summoning death once again rolled into the courthouse. Elizabeth Bouvia wanted to die, and she called a press conference to announce it and to ask for help. Bouvia was afflicted with cerebral palsy; she was quadriplegic, completely bedridden, and immobile. She could not feed herself or take care of any of her personal needs. She was in constant pain from arthritis, and had no financial means to support herself. She also had no family support. The prognosis was that her condition would never improve; she would always be in pain and always be completely dependent on others. She wanted to end her life, but was physically incapable of doing so because she had no use of her hands (*Bouvia v. Superior Court of Los Angeles* 179 Cal. App. 3d 1127 [1986]).

Initially, she asked hospital officials to help her starve to death, but the trial court intervened, and her request was denied. Later, she sought removal of a nasogastric feeding tube, but the trial court denied this request as well. She appealed and obtained an injunction from the Court of Appeal of California, which found that Bouvia had the right to refuse the feeding; that right was hers exclusively and could not be vetoed by medical professionals or the courts. It mattered not that removal of the tube would hasten her death. Moreover, the court found that such removal would not constitute suicide. The court found Bouvia to be competent to make decisions about her health and her future, and that as part of her right to privacy, she had the right to live out her life with dignity and peace according to her own choosing (*Bouvia v. Superior Court of Los Angeles*).

Discussions of death and dying continued to draw the attention of policy makers and the public. In 1987, the federal Office of Technology Assessment published *Institutional Protocols for Decisions about Life-Sustaining Treatments*, which sought to assist health providers in establishing protocols regarding withholding and withdrawal of life-sustaining treatments (Office of Technology Assessment 1987), and in 1988, the *Journal of the American Medical Association* published an anonymous article entitled, "It's Over, Debbie," which described a medical resident's decision to euthanize a young patient dying of ovarian cancer ("It's Over," 1988). Later that same year, national attention was riveted on the first-degree murder trial of Florida pathologist Peter Rosier, who openly admitted to providing what he thought would be a fatal dose of Seconal at the request of his cancer-ridden wife, and when the Seconal failed, he injected her with morphine.[11]

In 1990, the face of a retired Michigan pathologist was splashed across the front pages of American newspapers. On June 4, 1990, just 3 weeks before the U.S. Supreme Court would release its decision on withdrawing life-sustaining treatment, Jack Kevorkian was present at the suicide of an Alzheimer's patient, Janet Adkins. Kevorkian had built a "suicide machine" from spare parts found in hardware stores and garage sales, and Adkins flipped a switch to inject herself. Kevorkian continued to assist patients with their suicides, was charged with various crimes, and stood trial five times. Later, in November 1998, the CBS news program "60 Minutes" aired a videotape of Kevorkian giving a lethal injection to 52-year-old Thomas Youk, who had Lou Gehrig's disease. In April 1999, Kevorkian was convicted of second-degree murder and the delivery of a controlled substance to Youk and is currently serving time in prison (Public Broadcasting System 1998).

Others openly joined the debate about termination of care and assisted suicide. Dr. Timothy E. Quill published an account of his role in the death of a leukemia patient in the *New England Journal of Medicine*. He admitted not only prescribing a lethal dose of barbiturates, but explaining to the patient the amount needed to end her life. After her family called to say she had died, he went to her home, telephoned the medical examiner, and stated that the cause of death was acute leukemia (Quill 1991). The same year, Derek Humphrey published his "how to" book on suicide, *Final Exit*, which became a bestseller (Humphrey 1991). The American Medical Association joined the debate with a policy statement in 1992 opposing euthanasia or physician-assisted suicide (PAS), but supporting the "double effect" of palliative treatments that may "foreseeably hasten death" (American Medical Association 1992: 2233).

The Development of National Policies

The most important event of the early 1990s was the U.S. Supreme Court decision in *Cruzan v. Director, Missouri Department of Health* (1105. CT. 2841 [1990]). While *Quinlan* and *Bouvia* were important in terms of the public's discussion about withdrawing and withholding life-sustaining treatments, they were decided by state courts and therefore did not establish national legal precedence. National precedence was established with the Cruzan decision when the U.S. Supreme Court for the first time squarely addressed for the nation as a whole the issue of whether the U.S. Constitution grants persons a right to die.

Nancy Beth Cruzan, aged 25, was involved in a single-car accident on January 11, 1983, in rural Missouri, a state known for the prolife views of its public officials. The first emergency responders thought she was dead because they detected no pulse, and she was without oxygen for approximately 15 minutes before paramedics were able to restore her heartbeat and breathing. She never regained consciousness. Doctors diagnosed her as having severe brain injuries compounded by anoxia (lack of oxygen), and implanted a feeding tube through her abdomen. She lapsed into PVS and became a spastic quadriplegic. Doctors offered no hope for her recovery or a return to any level of consciousness, but she was able to breathe without a ventilator. Her care was paid for by the state, and she was a patient in a Missouri state hospital.

After 5 years in PVS, her parents requested that the feeding tube be removed, and that Nancy be allowed to die.[12] The hospital refused to honor the request without a court order, which the Cruzans subsequently obtained. The lower court's decision was then appealed to the Supreme Court of Missouri, which overturned it and rescinded the order for removal of the feeding tube (*Cruzan v. Harmon* 760 S.W. 2d 408, 410–442 [Mo. 1988] en bank). The Supreme Court of Missouri, while recognizing the patient's right to informed consent, based its decision on the Missouri Living Will statute, which "embodied a state policy strongly favoring the preservation of life" (*Cruzan v. Harmon*, pp. 419–420). Although Nancy's roommate had previously testified about a conversation in which Nancy had stated that she did not want to live as a "vegetable," the Supreme Court of Missouri found this testimony to be unreliable. It also rejected the contention that Nancy's family could be surrogate decision makers because there was no "clear and convincing" evidence about Nancy's views expressed when she was competent, as required by the Missouri Living Will statute (*Cruzan v. Harmon*).

The Cruzans appealed the Missouri Supreme Court decision to the U.S. Supreme Court, which heard arguments on December 6, 1989, and issued its decision on June 25, 1990. Although not a party to the litigation, the U.S. government filed an *amicus* (friend of the court) brief in support of the Missouri Supreme Court decision. The U.S. Supreme Court took the position that the fundamental issue to resolve was whether the State of Missouri could require "clear and convincing" evidence that Nancy, if competent, would want life-sustaining equipment withdrawn. There is a long tradition in the United States that competent

persons have constitutionally protected rights to have treatment withdrawn or withheld, and the Court upheld this tradition. At present, all
courts in the United States recognize these rights (Luce and Alpers 2001).

However, these same rights do not necessarily apply to an incompetent
person because an incompetent person is unable to make an informed
decision. The Court found that states are entitled to enact public policy
that requires clear and convincing evidence of the expression of the incompetent patient's wishes at a time when the patient was competent.
Specifically, states may require that for a surrogate to make the decision
to withdraw or withhold life-sustaining equipment, there must be "clear
and convincing" evidence that the surrogate's actions conform to the
expressed wishes made by the patient when he or she was competent
(*Cruzan v. Director*, pp. 2843, 2851–2852).

Moreover, the Court found that states are not required to consider a
patient's quality of life. Rather, the state may "assert an unqualified interest in the preservation of human life to be weighed against the constitutionally protected interests of the individual" (*Cruzan v. Director*,
p. 2853). Noting that an erroneous decision to withdraw life-sustaining
equipment is not correctible once the patient has died, the U.S. Supreme
Court affirmed the decision of the Supreme Court of Missouri. Although
Cruzan applied nationwide, in reality it only affected those states that
utilized the "clear and convincing" evidentiary standard, which at the
time were Missouri, New York, Maine, and Illinois (Gostin and Weir
1991).

Although they lost their appeal to the U.S. Supreme Court, the Cruzans continued their quest to allow Nancy to die. Six months after the
U.S. Supreme Court decision, the same trial judge who had originally
ordered the removal of Nancy's feeding tube issued a finding that
Nancy's parents had presented "clear and convincing" evidence that
she would not want to live in her present existence ("Right-to-die Case
Ends" 1990) after three former co-workers came forward stating that
Nancy had said specifically that she would not want to be kept alive in
a vegetative state. The State of Missouri did not appeal the ruling
(DeBenedictis 1991), and shortly thereafter, physicians at the Missouri
Rehabilitation Center discontinued the feedings. Nancy died on Decem-

ber 26, 1990, having become the most memorable actor in the debate about care for the terminally ill.

Shortly after the Cruzan decision was released, Congress enacted the Patient Self-Determination Act (PSDA) as part of the Omnibus Budget Reconciliation Act of 1990, with an effective starting date of December 1991. It required that health facilities inform patients about their right to refuse medical treatment and their right to formulate advance directives (living wills). Although all but six states already had laws providing for advance directives, fewer than 10 percent of Americans actually had executed them (Fletcher and White 1991).

Specifically, PSDA requires hospitals, nursing homes, home health care providers, and hospices receiving federal funds (i.e., Medicare or Medicaid funds), to: (1) provide written information to each individual concerning his or her rights under state law to make decisions concerning medical care, including the right to refuse medical care and the right to formulate an advance directive such as a written will;[13] (2) document in each individual's medical record whether he or she had executed an advance directive; (3) not condition care or discriminate in care based on whether the patient had executed an advance directive; (4) ensure compliance with the requirements of state law respecting advance directives; and (5) provide education for staff and community on issues relating to advance directives (Omnibus Budget Reconciliation Act of 1990. 101 P.L. 508; 104 Stat. 1288. Sec. 4206 [Nov. 5 1990]). In addition, the U.S. Department of Health and Human Services (DHHS) was required to mount a national campaign to educate the public about the provisions of PSDA and advance directives.

In 1995, the General Accounting Office (GAO) completed a study of the effectiveness of PSDA. Its findings indicated that both health care providers and DHHS had complied with PSDA requirements. Studies cited in the report, however, indicate that while well more than half of patients involved in the studies were aware of the opportunity to execute living wills, only 5 to 29 percent had done so (General Accounting Office 1995). A number of explanations were offered for these low rates. The timing of when patients are provided with information may be ineffective. Specifically, individuals need to learn about advance directives before their end-of-life planning is imminent. Waiting until they are admitted to the hospital or nursing home facility or when home care or hospice care are initiated is too late in the process; patients are usually seriously ill at this time and they and their families are overwhelmed with making other decisions.

Moreover, studies indicate that patients expect physicians to initiate these conversations, and physicians expect patients to initiate them. Physicians may be reluctant to discuss end-of-life care because they lack the knowledge or training on how to formulate advance directives; believe they are not necessary for young, healthy patients; are not compensated for the time involved with these discussions; or feel death is not an appropriate outcome of care. Other barriers include misunderstandings on the part of patients about advance directives, or the unavailability of friends or family members to act as surrogate decision makers. Some patients may be suspicious of advance directives and worry that it will limit their care (General Accounting Office 1995).

Even when advance directives have been executed, they may not always be adhered to. We have already discussed the fact that advance directives may have no impact on where a patient dies. Other difficulties include the fact that the advance directive may not be kept with the patient's chart or may not accompany a patient when he or she is transferred to another facility. Some advance directives lack specificity and clarity, and the patient and provider may not have discussed their terms. Moreover, the patient may not have really clarified in his or her own mind what treatments should be pursued during a terminal illness. Another complicating factor concerns family input. One study involving tube feeding found that physicians were more likely to follow family preferences than the provisions of advance directives, and some physicians follow their own values and choose not to implement the directives as written. Fear of litigation may also play a role in providers' decisions to follow or not follow the provisions of an advance directive (General Accounting Office 1995).

Bradley and Rizzo's 1994 study of nursing home patients finds a greater impact of PSDA than those studies cited by the GAO. Their study estimated that 34.7 percent of nursing home patients had advance directives in 1994 after the passage of the PSDA, compared with only 4.7

percent prior to its passage. Bradley and Rizzo's study also showed that execution of advance directives varied with demographic characteristics. Persons aged 76 to 90 years were more likely than those who were younger to have executed advance directives, well-educated persons more likely than the less educated, self-paying patients more likely than those with third-party coverage, and those admitted from hospitals more likely than those admitted from home (Bradley and Rizzo 1999).

Physician-Assisted Death

In 1994, a quarter century after publication of *On Death and Dying* triggered the public debate over terminal care, Oregon became the only state to legalize physician-assisted suicide (PAS) when voters enacted the Oregon Death with Dignity Act (DWDA) through a 51 percent approval at a citizen's initiative election.[14] Initially, implementation was delayed by a court injunction that was eventually lifted in October 1997. In November 1997, the Oregon legislature asked voters to repeal DWDA through the referendum process, but PAS was supported by 60 percent of voters (Oregon Department of Human Services 2003). Four years later in November 2001, U.S. Attorney General John Ashcroft issued an interpretation of the federal Controlled Substances Act that would prohibit physicians from prescribing controlled substances for purposes of physician-assisted suicide. As we go to press, that litigation is ongoing, and no court decision has been rendered. Thus, DWDA remains in effect.

In order to qualify for PAS, one must be a resident of Oregon, be at least 18 years old, have the ability to communicate regarding health care issues, and be diagnosed with a terminal illness that will lead to death within 6 months. The patient must make two oral requests to his or her physician 15 days apart and must also provide a written request signed by witnesses. The prescribing physician and a consulting physician must confirm the diagnosis and prognosis and must determine if the patient is "capable." If either physician believes the patient's judgment is impaired by psychiatric or psychological disorders, the patient must be referred for psychological examination. The prescribing physician must inform the patient of alternatives, including comfort care, hospice care, and pain control, and must request that the patient notify next of kin. Physicians must report all lethal medication prescriptions to the Oregon Department of Human Services (Oregon Department of Human Services 2003).

In 2002, 38 patients took their lives by utilizing PAS. This compares with 21 in 2001, 27 in 2000, 27 in 1999, and 16 in 1998. Compared with patients who died without physician assistance, PAS patients in 2002 were younger (a median age of 69 years), more likely to be divorced, well educated, had cancer (84 percent), and were enrolled in hospice programs (92 percent). More men used PAS than women, and all but one had health insurance. The reasons PAS patients cited for ending their lives included loss of autonomy, a decreasing ability to participate in activities that make life enjoyable, and losing control over bodily functions (Oregon Department of Human Services 2003). Ganzini et al. report that physicians granted approximately one out of six requests, and that one out of ten requests resulted in suicide (Ganzini et al. 2000; for additional analyses see Chin et al. 1999 and Ganzini et al. 2001).

As of this writing, no other state permits PAS, and federal funds may not be used for any type of assisted suicide, euthanasia, or mercy killing, or for promoting any of these (Assisted Suicide Funding Restriction Act of 1997. 105 P.L. 12; 111 Stat. 23 [April 30, 1997]). Despite this, studies indicate that physician- and nurse-assisted euthanasia exists in states other than Oregon. A survey of physicians in Washington State found that 12 percent of the respondents had received explicit requests for physician-assisted suicide; 24 percent of these patients were given prescriptions. An additional 4 percent of patients requested euthanasia, and 24 percent of these were given parenteral medication and died (Back et al. 1996).

A nationwide study of oncologists found that 16 percent participated in euthanasia or PAS. The most common method of assisted suicide was the prescription of drugs knowing that the patient intended to use them to commit suicide. Nearly 40 percent of responding oncologists feared prosecution (Emanuel et al. 1998). A study of critical care nurses showed that 17 percent had received euthanasia requests from patients or families, 16 percent had engaged in euthanasia or assisted suicide, and an additional 4 percent had hastened a patient's death by only pretending to provide life-sustaining treatment ordered by a physician (Asch 1996).

Physicians and nurses have good reason to fear prosecution. In 1997, the U.S. Supreme Court upheld criminal statutes that prohibited PAS in the states of Washington and New York in the companion cases of *Washington v. Glucksberg* and *Vacco v. Quill*. In each case, the plaintiffs were physicians and patients, the latter suffering from terminal and painful illnesses. The plaintiffs argued that prohibitions against PAS were unconstitutional because they violated the Fourteenth Amendment to the U.S. Constitution. Specifically, they argued that the existence of a liberty interest protected by the Fourteenth Amendment should extend to a personal choice by a mentally competent, terminally ill adult to commit suicide with the assistance of a physician (*Washington v. Glucksberg* 521 U.S. 702 [1997]).

In opinions written by Chief Justice Rehnquist, the Court upheld the constitutionality of the Washington and New York criminal bans on assisted suicide in finding that the statutes affect all citizens alike and do not infringe on fundamental rights or involve suspect classifications. The Court addressed the distinctions between death caused by withdrawing life-sustaining treatment and death caused by physician assistance. In the former, the patient dies from the underlying disease; in the latter, the patient is killed by the medication provided by the physician (*Vacco v. Quill* 521 U.S. 793 [1997]).

In *Glucksberg*, the Court noted the long tradition in Anglo-American common law of opposition to both suicide and assisting in suicide, and emphasized that nearly all states ban both. While reiterating its support for informed consent and the right of competent adults to refuse life-sustaining treatment, the Court found in *Glucksberg* that states had an interest in preventing suicide because people who consider suicide often suffer from depression or mental disorders and may change their minds if they are treated. Moreover, states have

an interest in protecting vulnerable groups—including the poor, the elderly, and disabled persons—from abuse, neglect, and mistakes.... We have recognized ... the real risk of subtle coercion and undue influence in end-of-life situations.... If physician-assisted suicide were permitted, many [patients] might resort to it to spare their families the substantial financial burden of end-of-life health-care costs.... The State's interest here goes beyond protecting the vulnerable from coercion; it extends to protecting disabled and terminally ill people from prejudice, negative and inaccurate stereotypes, and "societal indifference."... The

State's assisted-suicide ban reflects and reinforces its policy that the lives of terminally ill, disabled, and elderly people must be no less valued than the lives of the young and healthy, and that a seriously disabled person's suicidal impulses should be interpreted and treated the same way as anyone else's (*Washington v. Glucksberg*, 704).

The Supreme Court's position coincides with the position of the prestigious New York State Task Force on Life and the Law, which issued a policy statement in April 1997 opposing PAS. The task force points to physician failure to diagnose and treat mental illness and to effectively manage pain, and to the insufficient attention paid to the fears and feelings of abandonment in dying patients. It expresses concern about social inequality and the risks to the poor, elderly, isolated, members of minority groups, or those who lack access to good medical care. Particular concern is expressed for the disabled from the perspective that a physician's reaction may depend on his or her values about the disabled. Some patients may feel obligated to utilize PAS to relieve their loved ones from the burden of care, and patients may follow a physician's recommendations for PAS since patients tend to follow the recommendations of their physicians. Since PAS is less expensive than palliative care, there may be financial incentives to limit care. Finally, the task force points to the possible expansion of PAS to individuals who are not competent or are not terminally ill, and that overall, the possibility of developing effective regulation is impossible (New York State Task Force on Life and the Law 1997). It is worth noting, though, that most of these fears were not borne out by the Oregon experience.

The concurring opinions in *Glucksberg* and *Vacco* make important contributions to the debate in the United States regarding palliative care, even when such care causes death. In justifying her opposition to suicide and physician-assisted suicide, Justice O'Connor, a moderate on the Court, writes in *Glucksberg*:

[T]here is no need to address the question whether suffering patients have a constitutionally cognizable interest in obtaining relief from the suffering that they may experience in the last days of their lives. There is no dispute that dying patients ... can obtain palliative care, even when doing so would hasten their deaths (*Washington v. Glucksberg*, 737–738).

The issue of "terminal sedation" is directly addressed in *Vacco*. Citing the New York State Task Force report entitled "When Death Is Sought"

(New York State Task Force on Life and the Law 1994) outlining the ethical and professional acceptability of administering medication intended to alleviate pain even when that medication may hasten the patient's death, the Court acknowledged that even though states

may prohibit assisting suicide while permitting patients to refuse unwanted life-saving treatment, it may permit palliative care related to that refusal, which may have the foreseen but unintended "double effect" of hastening the patient's death (*Vacco v. Quill*, footnote 11).

Conclusions

Death policy in the United States is fairly well settled. Competent patients can refuse life-sustaining treatments. For incompetent patients, surrogate decision makers are to be appointed, and states may require "clear and convincing" evidence of what the patient's preferences would be if he or she were competent. The best mechanism for stating that preference is through execution of an advance directive. The national government sought to expand Americans' awareness of their right to execute such directives through passage of the Patient Self-Determination Act. However, advance directives are not a guarantee that a patient's preferences will be followed, and relatively few Americans have executed them. Despite studies showing that physicians and nurses nationwide participate in assisted suicide, such assistance is illegal, except in the State of Oregon. In 1969, Kubler-Ross initiated a discussion among the American people about the journey they and their families will take during terminal illnesses. Along that journey are many intersections. Through national and state statutory law and the decisions of national and state courts, particularly the U.S. Supreme Court, the journey and its path now have markers and directions.

Notes

1. For an in-depth analysis of the development of the health care industry from the eighteenth century to the late twentieth century, see Starr (1982).
2. Adjusted for differences in cost of living.
3. Reflects children under the age of 5 years.
4. Adjusted for differences in cost of living.

5. Medicare was established in 1965 to provide health insurance coverage for retired persons who had paid into the Social Security system. In 2001, Medicare covered 99.3 percent of those 65 years and older.

6. Medicaid, also established in 1965, provides health insurance coverage for low-income persons. It is funded and administered jointly by the federal government and the fifty state governments, and eligibility and coverage vary from state to state. In 2000, 12.4 million persons were covered by Medicaid for at least part of the year (see Mills, 2001).

7. For a comprehensive analysis of palliative care, see Doyle et al. (1998). For analysis of the nature of pain and patient suffering, see Cassel (1982), and for the role of the physician in relieving pain and assisting patients and families during terminal care, see Quill (2001).

8. For a comprehensive analysis of ethical and legal issues associated with American death policy, including decision-making procedures, informed consent, determination of incompetence, do-not-resuscitate statutes, advance directives, civil and criminal liability, futile treatments, and assisted suicide, see Meisel (1995). Updates are provided in annual supplements.

9. This is a coma in which the patient is profoundly nonresponsive and has no cognitive function, but appears to be awake.

10. The United States has a long tradition of informed consent. See *Schloendorff v. Society of the New York Hospital* (1211 N.Y. 125 [1914]) in which the Court of Appeals of New York ruled that every competent adult has the right to determine what shall be done with his body; a surgeon who performs an operation without consent, except in emergencies, commits assault. See also Gostin and Weir (1991).

11. At trial, it was learned that the dose of Seconal and the morphine injection were insufficient to cause Patricia Rosier's death, and unbeknownst to Dr. Rosier, Patricia's stepfather smothered her when he realized her attempt at suicide had failed. See "I Helped Her on Her Way" (1988).

12. It is important to differentiate between the types of life-sustaining equipment used for Quinlan and Cruzan. Quinlan's life was sustained by a respirator, but she received nutrition and hydration even after the respirator was removed. Cruzan was able to breathe without a respirator, but was receiving nutrition and hydration through a feeding tube. Those who opposed removal of the feeding tube characterized it as starving Cruzan to death.

13. This information is to be provided at the time of admission as an inpatient for hospitals and skilled nursing facilities. For home health care, the information must be provided prior to the patient coming under the care of the home health agency; and for hospice care, the information must be provided at the time of initial receipt of hospice care.

14. Some states, including Oregon, have procedures that allow citizens to enact statute law. The initiative procedure allows citizens to place a proposed law on the ballot and vote for or against its enactment. A referendum procedure allows

the state legislature to propose a law and place it on the ballot, and citizens are allowed to vote for or against it.

References

American Medical Association. 1992. "Decisions Near the End of Life." *Journal of the American Medical Association* 267 (16): 2229–2233.

Anderson, G. F., V. Petrosyan, and P. S. Hussey. 2002. Multinational Comparisons of Health Systems Data, 2002. Commonwealth Fund Website: www. cmwf.org. (accessed May 10, 2003).

Anderson, R. N. 2001. "Deaths: Leading Causes for 1999." *National Vital Statistics Reports* 49 (11). U.S. Department of Health and Human Services, Centers for Disease Control. Located at http://www.cdc.gov/nchs/data/nvsr/nvsr49/nvsr49_11.pdf (accessed May 25, 2003).

Asch, D. A. 1996. "The Role of Critical Care Nurses in Euthanasia and Assisted Suicide." *New England Journal of Medicine* 334 (21): 74–79.

Back, J. I., J. I. Wallace, H. E. Starks, and R. A. Pearlman. 1996. "Physician-Assisted Suicide and Euthanasia in Washington State: Patient Requests and Physician Responses." *Journal of the American Medical Association* 275 (12): 919–995.

Bradley, E. H., and J. A. Rizzo. 1999. "Public Information and Private Search: Evaluating the Patient Self-Determination Act." *Journal of Health Politics, Policy, and Law* 24 (2): 239–273.

Bradley, E. H., T. R. Fried, S. V. Kasl, D. V. Cicchetti, R. Johnson-Hurzeler, and S. M. Horwitz. 2000. "Referral of Terminally Ill Patients for Hospice: Frequency and Correlates." *Journal of Palliative Care* 16 (4): 20–26.

Cassel, C. K., J. M. Ludden, and G. M. Moon. 2000. "Perceptions of Barriers to High-Quality Palliative Care." *Health Affairs* 19 (5): 166–172.

Cassel, E. J. 1982. "The Nature of Suffering and the Goals of Medicine." *New England Journal of Medicine* 306 (11): 639–645.

Chin, A. E., K. Hedberg, G. K. Higginson, and D. W. Fleming. 1999. "Legalized Physician-Assisted Suicide in Oregon: The First Year's Experience." *New England Journal of Medicine* 340 (7): 577–583.

"Costs at the End of Life." 1999. *Managed Care Interface* 12 (8): 40–41.

Cristakis, N. A., and J. J. Escarce. 1996. "Survival of Medicare Patients after Enrollment in Hospice Programs." *New England Journal of Medicine* 355 (3): 172–178.

DeBenedictis, D. J. 1991. "Cruzan's Death Doesn't Still Debate." *American Bar Association Journal* March: 26–27.

Doyle, D., G. W. C. Hanks, and N. MacDonald, eds. 1998. *Oxford Textbook of Palliative Medicine*. Oxford: Oxford University Press.

Emanuel, E. J., E. R. Daniels, D. L. Fairclough, and B. R. Clarridge. 1998. "The Practice of Euthanasia and Physician-Assisted Suicide in the United States." *Journal of the American Medical Association* 280 (6): 507–513.

Fletcher, J. C., and M. L. White. 1991. "Patient Self-Determination Act to Become Law: How Should Institutions Prepare?" *BioLaw* 2 (46/47): S509–514 (special supp.).

Ganzini, L., H. D. Nelson, T. A. Schmidt, D. F. Kraemer, M. A. Delorit, and M. A. Lee. 2000. "Physicians' Experiences with the Oregon Death with Dignity Act." *New England Journal of Medicine* 342 (8): 557–563.

Ganzini, L., H. D. Nelson, M. A. Lee, D. F. Kraemer, T. A. Schmidt, and M. A. Delorit. 2001. "Oregon Physicians' Attitudes About and Experience with End-of-Life Care Since Passage of the Oregon Death with Dignity Act." *Journal of the American Medical Association* 285 (18): 2363–2369.

General Accounting Office. 1995. Patient Self-Determination Act: Providers Offer Information on Advance Directives but Effectiveness Uncertain. Report to the Ranking Minority Member, Subcommittee on Health, Committee on Ways and Means, U.S. House of Representatives, August 28.

Gostin, L., and R. F. Weir. 1991. "Life and Death Choices after Cruzan: Case Law and Standards of Professional Conduct." *Milbank Quarterly* 29 (1): 143–173.

Hogan, C., J. Lunney, J. Gabel, and J. Lynn. 2001. "Medicare Beneficiaries' Costs of Care in the Last Year of Life." *Health Affairs* 20 (4): 188–195.

Hospice Association of America. 2003. Fact or Fiction: Learning the Truth about Hospice. Website http://www.hospice-america.org (accessed May 11, 2003).

Humphrey, D. 1991. *Final Exit.* Secaucus, N.J.: Hemlock Society.

"I Helped Her on Her Way." 1988. *Newsweek,* November 7, p. 101.

Institute of Medicine. 2003. *Describing Death in America: What We Need to Know.* Washington, D.C.: Institute of Medicine.

"It's Over, Debbie." 1988. *Journal of the American Medical Association* 259 (2): 272.

Kubler-Ross, E. 1969. *On Death and Dying: What the Dying Have to Teach Doctors, Nurses, Clergy, and their Own Families.* New York: Simon and Schuster.

Levinsky, N. G., W. Yu, A. Ash, M. Moskowitz, G. Gazelle, O. Saynina, and E. J. Emanuel. 2001. "Influence of Age on Medicare Expenditures and Medical Care in the Last Year of Life." *Journal of the American Medical Association* 286 (11): 1349–1355.

Luce, J. M. and A. Alpers. 2001. "End-of-Life Care: What Do the American Courts Say?" *Critical Care Medicine* 29 (2): N40–N45 (supplement).

Meisel, A. 1995. *The Right to Die.* New York: Wiley.

Mills, R. J. 2001. Health Insurance Coverage: 2000. U.S. Census Bureau Website http://www.census.gov/prod/2001pubs/p60-215.pdf (accessed May 24, 2003).

New York State Task Force on Life and the Law. 1994. When Death Is Sought. N.Y. State Department of Health Website http://www.health.state.ny.us/nysdoh/provider/death.htm (accessed May 23, 2003).

New York Task Force on Life and the Law. 1997. *When Death is Sought (Supplement)*. N.Y. State Department of Health Website http://health.state.ny.us/nysdoh.taskfce/index.htm (accessed May 20, 2003).

Office of Technology Assessment. 1987. *Institutional Protocols for Decisions about Life-Sustaining Treatments*. Washington, D.C.: Government Printing Office.

Oregon Department of Human Services (ODHS). 2003. Fifth Annual Report on Oregon's Death with Dignity Act. ODHS Website http://www.ohd.hr.state.or.us/chs/pas/ar-intro.cfm#history (accessed May 18, 2003).

President's Commission for the Study of Ethical Problems in Medicine and Biomedical and Behavioral Research. 1983. *Deciding to Forego Life-Sustaining Treatment*. Washington, D.C.: Government Printing Office.

Pritchard, R. S., E. S. Fisher, J. M. Teno, S. M. Sharp, D. J. Reding, W. A. Knaus, J. E. Wennberg, and J. Lynn. 1998. "Influence of Patient Preferences and Local Health System Characteristics on the Place of Death." *Journal of the American Geriatrics Society* 46 (10): 1242–1250.

Public Broadcasting System. 1998. The Kevorkian Verdict. PBS Website http://www.pbs.org/wgbh/pages/frontline/kevorkian (accessed May 19, 2003).

Quill, T. E. 1991. "Death and Dignity: A Case of Individualized Decision Making." *New England Journal of Medicine* 324 (10): 691–694.

Quill, T. E. 2001. *Caring for Patients at the End of Life: Facing an Uncertain Future Together*. New York: Oxford University Press.

"Right-to-die Case Ends; Judge Says Feeding May be Stopped." 1990. *Minneapolis Star Tribune*, December 15, p. 1A.

Rollin, Betty. 1985. *Last Wish*. New York: Simon and Schuster.

Starr, Paul. 1982. *The Social Transformation of American Medicine: The Rise of a Sovereign Profession and the Making of a Vast Industry*. New York: Basic Books.

Teno, J. M., S. Weitzen, T. Wetle, and V. Mor. 2001. "Persistent Pain in Nursing Home Residents." *Journal of the American Medical Association* 285 (16): 2081.

Virnig, B. A., S. Kind, M. McBean, and E. Fisher. 2000. "Geographic Variation in Hospice Use Prior to Death." *Journal of the American Geriatric Society* 48 (9): 1117–1125.

World Health Organization. 2002. "The World Health Report 2002." World Health Organization Website www.who.int/whr/en/ (accessed May 9, 2003).

14

Summary: The State of End-of-Life Policy

Robert H. Blank

This chapter briefly describes the trends and patterns that emerge from the country summaries presented in this volume in terms of the wide disparities in attention and debate given end-of-life issues. In some cases, these chapters represent the first time this subject has been discussed in an English-language publication, and in several cases in any publication. The chapters on Brazil, China, India, Israel, Japan, Kenya, Taiwan, and Turkey, especially, provide illuminating insights into the importance of culture and religion, and demonstrate how narrowly this subject has been framed in the predominant literature. These findings reiterate the views of Macer (1998) and others that conventional Western-based bioethics must make clear its unique cultural foundations and thus its limits. Even in Western countries, however, these chapters illustrate how historical and cultural factors have created significant differences concerning end-of-life policy, and explain, for instance, why the Netherlands might embrace euthanasia while neighboring Germany as yet has not.

The studies presented here demonstrate that end-of-life policy across nations varies both in terms of substance and in refinement. Although all countries are addressing some of the issues raised in chapter 1, the importance of culture and economics cannot be overestimated when dealing with the profoundly emotional subject of death. "Death policy" is not an area that most medical professionals and politicians care to emphasize. For modern medicine, which is designed primarily to forestall it, death is often seen as a failure. Similarly, politicians are not anxious to risk their careers on what are often no-win, highly sensitive, and inflammatory issues with weighty moral dimensions. Despite this reluctance to set end-of-life policy, a multitude of factors has combined to place at least some of these issues on the political agendas of all the countries examined here. However, as vividly illustrated by the discussions in the preceding chapters, the framing of the issues varies significantly. Policies and concepts that in some countries enjoy widespread support are taboo elsewhere and are not even debatable.

Data on Dying

One of the first findings of most of the chapter authors was that systematic, accurate data on dying in their countries were not available. As a result, many of the quantitative questions posed in chapter 1 could not be answered. In some countries, there are no reliable data even on the number of deaths. In Brazil, for instance, Pessini concludes that there remains a cultural silence around death and few statistics are available. Turkey has no national statistics on dying and no data on the costs of dying. Likewise, India has no systematic data on the causes and costs of death. In Kenya, Wasunna suggests that the context of a highly paternalistic medical profession has worked counter to the collection of national statistics surrounding death. Li et al. found that the only way to study end-of-life policy in China was to focus on one province or city, in part for the lack of national data.

Israel, too, has few statistics and little research on death and dying, and, according to Amidror and Leavitt, it has no laws and little consensus. Even in legalistic Germany there are little empirical data on dying. Of all these countries, only Japan, Taiwan, the United Kingdom, and the United States systematically collect figures on the causes, costs, and even numbers of deaths nationally. Moreover, except for the United Kingdom and the United States, it was not possible to estimate the costs of dying. Even in the United Kingdom, where substantial records on death are kept, Ashcroft cautioned that the information is fragmented and of questionable reliability when it comes to estimating the cost of dying. This is not surprising in that the cost of dying is not readily identifiable in "health" statistics. As noted earlier, death is not what traditional medicine is about, even though it will be the ultimate result for all patients.

Where People Die

Some authors were better able to provide data on the proportion of people who die in various medical and nonmedical settings, although in most countries these numbers are based more on conjecture or rough estimates than on hard figures. The economic wealth and cultural heritage of the country appear to be important determinants of where people die. A key social factor is the strength of the extended family structure and the duty of family members to care for the dying person.

In most of the world and in a majority of our countries, most people die at home. In Turkey, for instance, Aksoy found that the duty of children to look after their parents, combined with limited access to life-support technologies, means that the vast majority of terminal patients die at home, even though no national statistics are available. Kenya, too, has a strong extended-family support system, a severely underfunded and stressed health care system, and very few available life-support systems. Therefore, as in Turkey, most deaths occur at home.

In India, another country with a poor medical infrastructure and a strong tradition of family responsibility, Pandya concludes that outside of urban areas, most people die at home. In urban areas, the middle and upper classes might go to hospitals or nursing homes, but since there are few intensive care units, the proportion that die there is insignificant. China, likewise, has a clear distinction between urban and rural areas. Although reliable estimates are not available, Li and associates suggest that the norm is for rural residents to die at home and urban residents in hospitals. In Taiwan, Chiu finds that an increasing number of terminal patients are dying in hospitals, especially in the urban areas where traditional culture has been diluted by Western values. However, the figures in 2000 still show that 58 percent die at home (80 percent in rural areas, 20 percent in urban) and only 35 percent in hospitals.

Only when we move to Western countries do we find majorities that die in hospitals. Simon estimates that about half the deaths in Germany occur in hospitals. Although national data on the deaths outside of hospitals are poor, a 1997 study from Rhineland-Palatinate found the following breakdown: 44 percent in hospitals, 13 percent in nursing homes, 40 percent at home, and 3 percent elsewhere. Similarly, despite its strongly rooted family tradition, in Japan a majority die in hospitals, although it must be noted that most "hospitals" in Japan are not large acute care medical centers, but smaller long-term facilities (Nakahara 1997).

Not surprisingly, the United Kingdom and the United States have the highest rates of in-hospital deaths. Relatively weak family support structures and the ready availability of life-support facilities have increased this rate over past decades. While most individuals in the United States express a desire to die at home, most do not. National estimates of deaths are 55 percent in hospitals, 25 percent at home, 9 percent in nursing homes, 9 percent in hospices, and 1 percent elsewhere. Merrick warns, however, that there is considerable variation in these figures across the United States and that the single best indicator is the availability of acute care in a specific locale; if acute care is available, it is used. Of all the countries examined here, the United Kingdom, with its national health service, appears to have the highest rates of death in a hospital setting. Based on his analysis, Ashcroft estimates that 65 percent of deaths occur in hospitals, 20 percent at home, 4 percent in hospices, and 8 percent in other communal establishments.

Palliative Care and Hospices

Closely linked to the question of where people die are palliative care and hospices, where a preponderance of palliative care takes place in some countries. Palliative care is quite limited and a relatively recent addition to end-of-life care in most countries, although it appears to be expanding. In Brazil, for instance, a national association for palliative care was founded in 1997, and there are at present only 29 palliative care centers spread across the entire population. Part of the reason for the paucity of work in pain management, according to Pessini, is a cultural view that one must suffer as part of life. In China, too, palliative care is a recent activity, but dedicated wards have been added in recent years. Taiwan has a recent (1990) but active hospice movement and has seen a relatively rapid expansion of inpatient and home-care programs. Pain management in Taiwan, however, remains inadequate, in part, according to Chiu, because of a cultural emphasis on Stoicism, under which patients often refuse pain medicine or cut prescribed dosages.

In Turkey, which has severely limited health care resources, palliative care is almost nonexistent. Pain management is inadequate, although recently some medical centers have established new departments dedicated to it. Moreover, a culture that sees it as a duty of children to look after their dying parents means most people die at home and that hospices do not exist except in a few nursing home settings. Similarly, Kenya has no pain management and palliative care services, although a charitable hospice movement has begun. In India there are a few charitable palliative care centers, but outside urban areas most people die at home without palliative resources.

In Germany there is a system of small, independent hospices as well as integrated palliative care centers, but they were relatively late in arriving. Home care offers pain therapy and symptom control but, as noted by Simon, since they are not covered by health insurance, hospice services are mostly volunteer based. According to ten Have, the relatively primitive state of palliative services in the Netherlands is partly a reflection of diminished options as a result of the heavy emphasis on euthanasia. However, specialized centers in pain control and management have been established in the past decade and interest in palliative care is on the rise in the Netherlands. Although Japan has had dedicated palliative care units since 1980, a cultural reluctance to use them means that less than 1 percent of deaths overall occur in a hospice, and, according to Macer, pain management in Japan remains inadequate.

In contrast, other countries have more extensive palliative care facilities and services. Israel has a well-established institutional and home-care hospice system. The United Kingdom was the birthplace of the hospice movement although it remains overwhelmingly charitable and thus a low priority for the National Health Service. The United States also has a well-established hospice system that emerged with cancer patients in the 1960s and expanded to AIDS patients in the 1980s, although overall the use of hospices has been low. As Merrick suggests, however, owing to the increase in managed care, the use of hospices as a less expensive option for dying is on the rise. Despite this, pain management and palliative care are underfunded in the United States.

Advance Directives

The legal status of advance directives, too, varies widely across these countries, but even in those countries that formally allow them, use rates remain low. Indian law does not recognize advance directives of any type. In Kenya they are seldom used, and in some African cultures they are rejected because they are seen as inviting death. Turkish law allows advance directives, but they are not binding and are often ignored, according to Aksoy. In contrast, do-not-resuscitate (DNR) orders are illegal in Turkey, but they are practiced. Likewise, advance directives are rare in China, and in Israel advance directives have unclear status and are seldom used.

Although Japanese statutes allow living wills, they are rare, and less than 1 percent of patients die with some form of advance directive. While German law recognizes advance directives, court approval is necessary in each case, and as a result few people bother to have one. In Taiwan, the process for advance directives was formalized by the Natural Death Act of 2000. According to the act, terminally ill patients have the right to make a living will or appoint a durable power of attorney that can be executed after two doctors certify that the patient suffers from a terminal illness. Despite the act, actual use in Taiwan remains very low according to Chiu.

The Netherlands has a special procedure through which a patient can request euthanasia before becoming incompetent. Although a variety of advance directives are legal in the United Kingdom, their use is not widespread. Of all the countries examined here, the United States stands alone in terms of attention paid to advance directives, perhaps because of the emphasis on individual rights and a highly litigious system, but even in the United States, advance directives are utilized in a very small proportion of deaths.

Euthanasia

There remains considerable confusion over even the definition of euthanasia in many countries, and as a concept it is considerably less obvious than some Western observers assume. Although assisted suicide remains illegal in most countries, including the Netherlands, in many countries there has been a trend toward acceptance or at least tolerance of other forms of euthanasia, particularly the withholding of medical technologies at the request of a competent patient. Again, culture and the sophistication and availability of medical technologies in a country appear to be major influences.

In Kenya, for example, there are few facilities for life support, and euthanasia is illegal. Wasunna, however, notes that there recently has been a surge in requests for doctor-assisted suicide because of the AIDS epidemic. Similarly, in Turkey euthanasia of any form is unlawful. Although Turkey is a secular state, its 95 percent Muslim population guarantees that the Islamic prohibition against euthanasia is embedded in criminal law, according to Aksoy. As in Kenya and Turkey, euthanasia in India is against the law in all circumstances. Moreover, there has been little public debate over a right to die. In all three of these countries, the absence of life-sustaining intensive care facilities at the end of life means that passive euthanasia as defined in the West is a near-meaningless concept since there is nothing to withdraw or withhold.

Israel is an interesting case in that there is neither written law nor obligatory unwritten rules regarding euthanasia. According to Amidror and Leavitt, the result is that end-of-life policy varies from one medical center to the next and often from one ward to another in the same center. Although it is unclear if a patient has the right to refuse life-sustaining treatment, there is increasing openness to withholding (but not withdrawing) such treatment, although it remains a minority opinion. The authors note that any form of active euthanasia is unlikely to ever be acceptable in Israel, although high doses of morphine that result in death might be given for pain relief.

In Japan, a medical treatment used to remove or reduce pain that might also cause premature death is lawful, but only if the patient suffers from an incurable disease, the pain is unbearable, and the patient consents. Macer notes that anyone assisting death is liable to be punished under law, but the courts have shown leniency, especially for family members who do so. According to Pessini, a strong tradition of absolute respect for human life in Brazil has meant that even with a change in the code in 1988 to include quality-of-life considerations, there are no national laws that protect withholding of treatment or DNR orders. Despite this, in 1999 São Paulo State enacted a law that gives individuals the right to refuse painful or extraordinary attempts to prolong life.

As in these other countries, active euthanasia is illegal in China and forbidden in clinical practice. China has no formal euthanasia law and there are no clear standards or indicators for withdrawing therapy. Moreover, while there has been some discussion in government, to date there has been no formal law on passive euthanasia. Although active euthanasia also remains illegal in Taiwan, some argued for it during the 6-year debate over the drafting of the Natural Death Act of 2002. The act did formalize procedures for withdrawal of life-support systems, although as Chiu points out, implementation of the law has not been without difficulty.

In Germany, the courts in the 1980s ruled that there is no obligation to sustain life and that life-support treatment can be withheld or withdrawn if the will of the patient is known. Moreover, the prescription of drugs to reduce pain is allowed even if it leads to death. Active euthanasia in Germany is prohibited by criminal law, although the status of assisted suicide policy is more complicated. A physician cannot be punished for assisting in the suicide of a patient by supplying drugs as long as the death does not occur in his or her presence. For Simon this legal situation makes assisted suicide a difficult option because it forces the person administering the euthanasia to leave the dying person at the end in order to escape prosecution.

In the United Kingdom, voluntary passive euthanasia is widely accepted and practiced. In contrast, as borne out by highly publicized court cases described by Ashcroft, active euthanasia in any form remains a criminal offense. Despite this legal status, however, in practice it is not clear-cut and there have been few prosecutions for assisted suicide. In these cases, the verdicts have been especially lenient for family members convicted of killing a loved one. As usual, there has been considerable variation across the United States. However, as discussed by Merrick, a series of high-profile court rulings and an active right-to-die movement have resulted in the legalization of voluntary passive euthanasia through the withholding or withdrawal of life-sustaining technologies. Active euthanasia is illegal in all but one of the fifty states, but like the United Kingdom, in practice prosecution has been limited in other states. Oregon has been the only state to legalize physician-assisted suicide, but under very strict controls; the number killed has been under fifty annually (thirty-eight in 2000).

Much attention has been directed to the euthanasia policy of the Netherlands, but ten Have argues that it remains controversial and is still not an established, normal practice. Although the Termination of Life on Request and Assisted Suicide Act does legalize such actions when they are performed by a physician, the Dutch government insists that the law does not legalize active euthanasia, but merely provides a punishment exclusion ensuring that physicians will not be prosecuted. So even in what some international observers see as an unambiguous case of active euthanasia, the situation remains unsettled.

Overall then, these countries present a wide range of responses to the broad issue of euthanasia. As many of the authors point out, this is an area where there is substantial inconsistency between the formal law and actual practice, particularly as related to the withholding and withdrawal of treatment and the use of pain-killing drugs to relieve suffering. Even in those countries with strong cultural objections to euthanasia and with Stoic traditions, there are indications that clinical practice, particularly that related to the use of drugs to relieve suffering, often does not correspond to either the law or the culture.

Definition of Death

For American observers, brain death as a concept is widely accepted and often assumed to be the universal definition of death. This review of other countries, however, shows that the debate over brain death and its connections and implications for organ donations has been at best muted elsewhere. Of those countries where it has been an issue, only in the United Kingdom and the United States is brain death widely accepted and used as the basis for organ removal. In Kenya, there is no recognition of brain death, and organs cannot be transplanted. Similarly, in Israel there is a general refusal to accept the concept of brain death and thus there is a very low rate of organ transplantation.

Although brain death is defined by law in India, most families refuse to accept it and choose to wait for cardiovascular death to occur. However, there is strong support for organ removal since under the Hindu and Buddhist traditions the body means nothing at death. In Japan there has been a heated debate over brain death and organ transplantation, and although the laws are changing, there remains little public acceptance of brain death, and very few transplants are performed. Brazil, on the other hand, has seen increased acceptance of brain death and a transplant number second only to the United States, even though a law to require presumed consent designed to increase organ donation rates was repealed after strong public opposition.

Policy Arenas and the Question of Convergence

In addition to facilitating this comparison of the many substantive areas surrounding the end of life, the analyses here demonstrate considerable variation in the role of governments in end-of-life decision making. There is also wide divergence in these countries over the stage of debate on specific death issues as well as where this debate takes place—among government policy makers, the medical profession, commissions or committees, academics, or a public forum. Moreover, while a few governments like those of the Netherlands and Taiwan have passed specific legislation, in most others end-of-life decision making has largely been left to the medical profession or, as in the United Kingdom and the United States, handled through court decisions in particular cases. In a few countries, ethics committees are active in the decision process, but overall the Western emphasis on such mechanisms has seen limited applicability elsewhere.

Although economic pressures and the desire to reduce pain and suffering appear to be breaking down some past restrictions, particularly as related to pain management and the withholding or withdrawing of life-support systems, overall convergence appears very limited. Even in those areas that some observers might see as more straightforward, such as hospice and palliative care, brain death, and advance directives, there is nothing approaching convergence across these countries. On euthanasia, especially, there is unlikely to ever be convergence. Death-related issues are too intense and culturally sensitive to expect a convergence to the Western, largely U.S.-driven, norms despite the difficult resource allocation questions surrounding the end of life and aging populations that cross national boundaries.

Even more so than in other areas of medicine, issues at the end of life highlight the importance of religion and culture, as well as the role of the family and the social structure. In most countries examined here, even the Western ones, there is still fervent opposition to change on these issues among large segments of the population and health care professions. The accounts of these twelve countries clearly demonstrate how contentious these issues are. In many countries, there remains the feeling that death is a highly personal matter, not something to be publicly discussed, much less made a matter of public policy. As discussed here, however, in all countries these issues are finding their way onto the public policy agenda and as such will increasingly become continuous and unremitting political issues for the twenty-first century. We hope that this book will lead to more in-depth comparative studies of end-of-life issues in these and other countries.

References

Macer, D. 1998. *Bioethics in Asia*. Christchurch, New Zealand: Eubios Ethics Institute.

Nakahara, T. 1997. "The Health System of Japan." In M. W. Raffel, ed. *Health Care and Reform in Industrialized Countries*. University Park, PA: Pennsylvania State University Press.

Contributors

Sahin Aksoy, M.D., Ph.D., Department of Medical Ethics, Harran University Faculty of Medicine, Sanliurfa, Turkey

Tali Amidror, R.N., B.S.N., Neonatal Intensive Care Unit, Hadassah Hospital, Jerusalem, Israel

Richard Ashcroft, Ph.D., Department of Primary Health Care and General Practice, Imperial College of Science, Technology, and Medicine, London, United Kingdom

Robert H. Blank, Ph.D., Brunel University, Uxbridge, United Kingdom

Tai-Yuan Chiu, M.D., M.H.Sci., Department of Family Medicine and Social Medicine, College of Medicine and Hospital, National Taiwan University, Taipei, Taiwan

Ole Döring, Ph.D., Faculty for East Asian Studies, Bochum University, Hamburg, Germany

Frank J. Leavitt, Ph.D., The Center for Asian and International Bioethics, Ben Gurion University of the Negev, Beer Sheva, Israel

Fu Li, Capital University of Medical Sciences, Beijing, China

Li Yiting, Professor of Medical Ethics, Capital University of Medical Sciences, Beijing, China

Liu Fang, Medical Morality Education, Capital University of Medical Sciences, Beijing, China

Darryl Macer, Ph.D., Institute of Biological Sciences, University of Tsukuba, Tsukuba City, Japan

Janna C. Merrick, Ph.D., Department of Government and International Affairs, University of South Florida, Tampa, Florida, USA

Sunil K. Pandya, M.D., Neurosurgery Department, Jaslok Hospital and Research Center, Mumbai, India

Léo Pessini, Ph.D., Center for Bioethics, St. Camillus College, São Paulo, Brazil

Alfred Simon, Ph.D., German Academy for Ethics in Medicine, Goettingen, Germany

Su Baoqi, Center for Bioethics, Beijing Union Medical College, Beijing, China

Henk ten Have, Ph.D., Professor of Medical Ethics, University of Nijmegen, Nijmegen, The Netherlands

Angela Wasunna, L.L.B., L.L.M., The Hastings Center, Garrison, New York, USA

Index